W9-AVR-733

# Dr. Earl Mindell's Unsafe at Any Meal

## How to Avoid Hidden Toxins in Your Food

Earl Mindell, R.Ph., Ph.D.
*and* Hester Mundis

**Contemporary Books**
*Chicago New York San Francisco Lisbon London Madrid Mexico City Milan New Delhi San Juan Seoul Singapore Sydney Toronto*

**Library of Congress Cataloging-in-Publication Data**

Mindell, Earl.
     Unsafe at any meal : how to avoid hidden toxins in your food / Earl Mindell with
Hester Mundis.—Rev. and updated
          p.     cm.
     Includes bibliographical references and index.
     ISBN 0-658-02115-X
     1. Nutrition.     2. Food—Toxicology.     3. Natural foods.     I. Mundis, Hester.
II. Title.

RA784 .M5148     2002
613.2—dc21                                                         2001058223

# *Contemporary Books* 𝄐

### A Division of The *McGraw·Hill* Companies

Copyright © 2002 by Earl Mindell, Ph.D. and Hester Mundis. All rights reserved. Printed in the
United States of America. Except as permitted under the United States Copyright Act of
1976, no part of this publication may be reproduced or distributed in any form or by any
means, or stored in a database or retrieval system, without the prior written permission of the
publisher.

1 2 3 4 5 6 7 8 9 10   DOC/DOC   1 0 9 8 7 6 5 4 3 2

ISBN 0-658-02115-X

This book was set in Garamond MT by Reider Publishing Services
Printed and bound by R. R. Donnelley—Crawfordsville

Cover design: Monica Baziuk
Cover photograph: Burke/Triolo Productions/Getty Images

McGraw-Hill books are available at special quantity discounts to use as premiums and sales
promotions, or for use in corporate training programs. For more information, please write to
the Director of Special Sales, Professional Publishing, McGraw-Hill, Two Penn Plaza, New
York, NY 10121-2298. Or contact your local bookstore.

This book is printed on acid-free paper.

*This book is dedicated to Gail, Alanna, Evan,*
*my parents and families, my friends and associates,*
*and to the continuing happiness*
*and healthiness of people everywhere.*

# Contents

1. Why You Still Can't Judge a Food by Its Label • 2. Where Did Those Percentages Come From? • 3. What Must Appear on a Food Label? • 4. What's Allowed to Go Unmentioned Is Unforgivable • 5. "Labelese": How General Terms Can Be Particularly Confusing • 6. Yes, What You Don't Know *Can* Harm You • 7. Basic "Labelese" for Beginners in Search of Better Health • 8. Label Highs and Lows at a Glance • 9. How Fresh Is "Fresh"? • 10. What Manufacturers Can Say and What They Mean • 11. How Natural Is "Organic"? • 12. Check Those Serving Sizes • 13. How to Find Hidden Ingredients • 14. Foods That Don't Have to Tell • 15. Coping with Invisible Ingredients • 16. What's in a Flavor? • 17. Flavoring Labeling Translated • 18. Those Mysterious "Spices" • 19. Are You Getting the Right USDA Grades? •

# Acknowledgments

I WISH TO express my deep and lasting appreciation to my friends and associates who have assisted me in the preparation of this book, especially J. Kenney, Ph.D., Harold Segal, Ph.D., Bernard Bubman, R.Ph., Mel Rich, R.Ph., Sal Messineo, R.Ph., Alan Khasin, R.Ph., Ph.D., Arnold Fox, M.D., Dennis Huddleson, M.D., Stewart Fisher, M.D., David Velkoff, M.D., Rory Jaffee, M.D., Vickie Hufnagel, M.D., Donald Cruden, O.D., Joel Strom, D.D.S., Nathan Sperling, D.D.S., Ray Faltinsky, Kevin Fournier, Rick Handel, Linda Chae, Morten Weidner, Ph.D., Carol Coleman Gerber, Jane Lyke, and Hester Mundis.

I would also like to thank the Center for Food Safety and Applied Nutrition, the American Medical Association, the American Dietetic Association, the United Fresh Fruit and Vegetable Association, the Society for Nutrition Education, the Prince-Pottenger Nutrition Foundation, the National Dairy Council, the United States Department of Agriculture, the U.S. Environmental Protection Agency, the American Cancer Society, Ron VanWarmer, and Richard Curtis, without whom a project of this scope could never have been completed.

# Preface

EVERY DAY people make choices that will affect their health and their lives—choices about what they are or are not going to eat. Most of us choose foods that we like best and, hopefully, are the best for us (or at least not harmful if consumed in moderation). We base our decisions on the health and nutrition information we've received from food labels, the media, and the recommendations and assurances of numerous government agencies. Unfortunately, despite the current long-overdue revisions in labeling, packaging, and marketing laws, much of this information remains confusing, misleading, and far too often dangerously inaccurate. Because of this, millions of Americans today are totally unaware of how many of the foods they rely on cannot be trusted—and that they may be unwittingly undermining their health at every meal.

Since 1987, when the first version of my book appeared, the food industry and regulatory agencies have "cleaned up their act" to a certain extent. But that progress is far from satisfactory or safe when more than 425 people die annually from food tainted with *Listeria monocytogenes* and there are over seventy-six million cases of food-borne illness each year; when so many antibiotics are being given to farm animals that ten thousand people die each year because of antibiotic-resistant strains of bacteria; when cheeses wrapped in deli-counter plastic contain high levels of toxins; when the USDA allows poultry processors to dump chicken carcasses into tubs of water and the chickens leave the baths more contaminated than when they entered; when two out of five peaches harbor potentially dangerous levels of pesticide residue; when nearly three thousand additives that can cause everything from asthma and headaches to miscarriages, heart problems, and cancer are still being concealed in our diets.

It is no coincidence that despite all the remarkable medical advances we've made in recent years, rates of cancer, Alzheimer's disease, multiple sclerosis, diabetes, and heart disease have steadily increased and are now at the highest point in history. It's also no coincidence that despite all the no-fat, low-fat foods on the market, Americans are fatter than ever (one in every four is obese), and the single biggest killer after smoking is excess weight.

At a time when fears of mad cow disease are evident and genetically modified food ingredients are hidden, when the average American is consuming over 155 pounds of sugar and 15 pounds of salt annually without knowing it, when "natural flavors" can be chemical concoctions without label disclosure, and people continue to think of a bowl of pasta as a portion, the need for a health defense guide has never been greater.

The purpose of this book is to show you how to navigate the nutritional minefield of hidden hazards in the foods we eat, the meals we serve, and the water we drink in a realistic way. I say *realistic* because there is no single diet that is ideal for everyone. I don't expect meat-loving readers to suddenly renounce charcoal-broiled steaks for veggie burgers, or pretend that kids who are hooked on fast foods can be easily switched to whole grains. What I have done, therefore, is to explain the health risks and, wherever possible, suggest trade-offs that can diminish these risks.

Each section is numbered and cross-referenced to help you easily locate information related to a particular food, additive, or dietary need. I've included detailed information on what to look—and look out—for. I've also stated name brands, explained ways to spot and avoid genetically modified foods, and individualized, to the best of my ability, cautions pertaining to foods, drugs, and nutrients by providing warning notices for high-risk consumers and alternatives for those who might have any medical problem or special health condition.

My supplement suggestions in *all* instances are *not* prescriptive. They are offered only as suggestions and should be discussed with your doctor. No book is or ought to be regarded as a substitute for professional care.

This book has been designed to help you help yourself. I've attempted to lift the "grease curtain" on convenience foods and foods you never thought were anything but wholesome; blow the whistle on seditious salt and sugar traps; shake you with the reality of deadly chemicals that might be pouring from your tap or hidden in your snacks, booze, health foods, breakfast, lunch, and dinner. It is my sincere hope that in pointing out all that you have not been told (or never realized) about what you've been eating, I will enable you to make the right food choices, choices that will help you and your family live longer, healthier, and happier lives.

EARL L. MINDELL, R.Ph., Ph.D.

# A Note to the Reader

ALL FOOD and supplement regimens discussed throughout this book are *recommendations, not prescriptions, and are not intended as medical advice.* Before making any changes in your current diet or starting any supplemental program, check with your physician or a nutritionally oriented doctor—especially if you have a specific physical problem or are taking any medication.

All brand name nutritional information in the book is accurate as of November 2001.

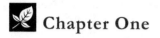 Chapter One

# The Lowdown on Labels

## 1. Why You Still Can't Judge a Food by Its Label

Unless you know what to look for, food labels can be inadequate, confusing, and dangerously misleading sources of dietary information. In 1990, the Nutrition Labeling and Education Act (NLEA) went into effect. The U.S. Department of Agriculture (USDA) and the Food and Drug Administration (FDA) helped design long-overdue requirements for labels so that consumers would have clear, nonmisleading information about the foods they eat—and be able to understand their relative significance in the context of a total daily diet. To do this, these agencies devised the Daily Values and the percent Daily Values system, based on a diet containing 2,000 calories a day.

This is a step in the right direction. But unless you understand *where* these percentages come from, *how* they vary if you're eating more or less than 2,000 calories a day, and *why* even if a product claims to provide 100 percent of a nutrient you might not be getting it, you still can be nutritionally sandbagged.

## 2. Where Did Those Percentages Come From?

RDIs (Reference Daily Intakes) for vitamins and minerals, and DRVs (Daily Reference Values) for protein, fat, and carbohydrates are the basis for calculating percent Daily Values. (The RDIs have replaced the term *U.S. RDAs,* [Recommended Daily Allowances], but are still based on the old National Academy of Sciences RDAs [Recommended Dietary Allowances], which I and many other leading nutritionists feel remain woefully inadequate.)

Stress and illness, past or present, affect each person's nutritional requirements differently. In other words, just because a product claims to provide 100 percent of your DV for a nutrient doesn't necessarily mean that *you* are getting it—or that it's a sufficient amount for *your* individual needs. (See section 31 for my basic supplement regimen.)

The 2,000 calories established as the reference for calculating percent Daily Values was chosen because it approximates the maintenance calorie requirements of postmenopausal women, the group most often targeted for weight reduction.

**One nutrient percentage does not fit all!**

Whatever the calorie level, DRVs, which were established for the energy-producing nutrients fat, saturated fat, total carbohydrate (including fiber), and protein—as well as for cholesterol, sodium, and potassium, which do not contribute calories—are always calculated as follows:

- Fat based on 30 percent of calories
- Saturated fat based on 10 percent of calories
- Carbohydrate based on 60 percent of calories
- Protein based on 10 percent of calories—the DRV for protein applies only to adults and children over the age of four; RDIs for protein for special groups have been established
- Fiber based on 11.5 g of fiber per 1,000 calories

DRVs for total fat, saturated fat, cholesterol, and sodium, because of current health recommendations, represent the uppermost limit considered desirable. They are:

- Total fat: less than 65 g
- Saturated fat: less than 20 g
- Cholesterol: less than 300 mg
- Sodium: less than 2,400 mg

## 3. What Must Appear on a Food Label?

All food labels now must contain the following information:

- Common name of the product
- Name and address of the product's manufacturer
- Net contents in terms of weight, measure, or count
- Ingredient list (in descending order of predominance and weight)
- Serving size
- Nutrition facts that identify the quantities of specified nutrients and food constituents for a single serving

### KEEP IN MIND

1 g of fat = 9 calories
1 g of protein = 4 calories
1 g of carbohydrate = 4 calories
1 g of alcohol = 7 calories

## 4. What's Allowed to Go Unmentioned Is Unforgivable

Considering that such prominent agencies as the USDA, the FDA, and the FTC (Federal Trade Commission) are in charge of food labeling, it's unforgivable that:

- Specific identification of *all* flavorings, spices, fats, and oils is not mandatory.

- There is no mandatory labeling in America for bioengineered foods or ingredients, genetically modified (GM) foods, or foods containing genetically modified organisms (GMOs). (See section 35.)
- Not all additives must be listed.
- It is not mandatory for manufacturers to label prominently foods containing peanuts, eggs, soy, wheat, and certain other possibly life-threatening allergens.
- All products need not disclose the presence of specific artificial coloring unless the coloring has been *proven* hazardous to health (for instance, yellow dye FD&C No. 5, tartrazine).
- Sulfites, preservative chemicals implicated in more than a dozen deaths, do not have to be listed on all product labels.

I also think it's unforgivable that despite the NLEA, foods can continue to legally claim "no preservatives" and still contain them because they are added before processing, and that products labeled "salt free" can still contain sodium, but that's another story. This is called "labelese" and is about the deceptive but legal liberties manufacturers are still allowed; it's not a pretty tale.

**About 150 Americans die each year from food allergies, usually from unknowingly eating foods with peanuts or tree nuts.**

## 5. "Labelese": How General Terms Can Be Particularly Confusing

The Food and Drug Administration (FDA) and the United States Department of Agriculture (USDA) have established "Definitions" and "Standards of Identity" as references for food labeling. These regulations determine such things as minimum standards of composition for common foods, what additives need not be listed because they're Generally Recognized As Safe (GRAS) (see section 25), and when and what generalized terms may be used in place of specific ingredients.

4

THE LOWDOWN ON LABELS

Also, under the NLEA, nutrient requirement claims may only be made if the FDA has spelled out the criteria for these claims. Their purpose—an admirable one—is to simplify label reading while protecting consumers from being ripped off, nutritionally and financially. But the creation of the "Nutrition Facts" panel—with its various mandatory and voluntary components—has resulted in more ways for manufacturers to hide ingredients that might make their product less appealing to buyers, or make it seem more nutritious than it actually is.

Though only safe ingredients are permitted for generalized categorization, what is safe for some people is not safe for all—and what is considered safe today might be proven otherwise tomorrow.

## 6. Yes, What You Don't Know *Can* Harm You

Without a clear understanding of "labelese," you could be seriously undermining your health right now and not know it.

Misinterpreting food label information can:

- *Sabotage physical and emotional fitness*
  Cause fatigue, insomnia, headaches, stomachaches, nausea, rashes, diarrhea, dizziness, depression, mood swings, breathing difficulties, and more. (See section 28.)
- *Decrease or alter the effectiveness of medications*
  Analgesics, antibiotics, anticoagulants, anticonvulsants, antidiabetics, antidyskinetics, antihistamines, antieoplastics, appetite suppressants, bronchial dilators, cardiovascular preparations, oral contraceptives, decongestants, diuretics, sedatives, thyroid drugs, tranquilizers, and more. (See section 142.)

## 7. Basic "Labelese" for Beginners in Search of Better Health

The following is a guide to the most commonly misinterpreted labels, explaining what they do—and do not—mean, and noting consumers who should be particularly aware of them.

## LABELS MOST LIKELY TO MISLEAD

**Diet or Dietetic**  This does *not* mean the food is carbohydrate free. Nor does it mean that it's necessarily low in sugar, sucrose, sodium, or even fat. *Dietetic* is a general term meaning that one or more of the ingredients usually found in a similar product have been replaced with other ingredients. Unless the label clearly states that the product is intended for use in a specific type of restricted diet, it generally isn't.

**CONSUMER ALERT**  Asthmatics, allergic individuals, diabetics, hyperactive children, dieters.

**Light or Lite**  This means either one-third fewer calories than the regular product (which could have a lot more than you thought) or at least half the fat of the comparison food. (If 50 percent or more of the calories come from fat, the reduction must be 50 percent of the fat of the comparison food.) But "light" can also mean light in syrup density or color. Though the label must state this, consumers often just assume that all light—or lite—products are low in calories. "Light" can also mean that the sodium content of a food has been reduced by 50 percent.

**CONSUMER ALERT**  Dieters, hypertensives.

**Lean and Extra Lean**  When used on meat, poultry, or seafood, *lean* means that there are less than 10 g of fat, 4.5 g of saturated fat, and 95 mg of cholesterol in each 100 g serving. *Extra lean,* for meat, poultry, or seafood, means that there are less than 5 g of fat, 2 g of saturated fat, and 95 mg of cholesterol in each 100 g serving. (A brand name containing the word *lean,* such as Lean Cuisine, can continue using its name even if it doesn't meet this criterion, if it was in use prior to November 27, 1991.)

**CONSUMER ALERT**  Dieters, anyone with cardiovascular or gastrointestinal problems.

**Light Beer or Wine**  Labeling of beer and wine (see sections 91 to 94) is regulated by the Bureau of Alcohol, Tobacco, and Firearms (BATF). A light beer will usually have one-third fewer calories than its regular counterpart, but not always. Sometimes, the word *light* refers to other factors, such as the beer's taste, color, or body. The same is basically true for wine. A "light" wine can contain no more than 14 percent alcohol, but not many table wines do. And since there are no requirements for how few calories a "light" beer or wine contains, weight-watching consumers can be easily left in the dark.

**CONSUMER ALERT**  Dieters.

**Low Calorie**  A food labeled "low calorie" can have no more than 40 calories per serving. This is fair—it is the serving sizes that aren't. Because manufacturers can change them, and do, what might formerly have been a single serving could now be two. (See section 12.)

**CONSUMER ALERT**  Dieters.

**Low Fat**  Any product that claims to be low fat cannot have more than 3 g of fat per serving. The danger of confusion here is that although labels must list the calories from fat that are in a serving, listing the calories from saturated fat is not mandatory. On the other hand, it is mandatory to list the percentage of fat and saturated fat in the serving, but, unfortunately, not mandatory to disclose the amounts of polyunsaturated and monounsaturated fat. (Keep in mind that trans-fats—fats that are produced when vegetable oils are partially hydrogenated to stiffen them for use as margarine or shortening—have been found to be potentially bad for the heart and arteries. See section 54.)

**CONSUMER ALERT**  Dieters, anyone with cardiovascular or gastrointestinal concerns.

**Low Sodium**  A low-sodium product can have no more than 140 mg per serving. This in itself is fine, but it can mislead consumers who are unaware that today's serving sizes might be much smaller than former ones, as is the case with many popular soups and snacks. A bag of microwave popcorn, which far too many people feel is a single serving, is generally three servings. So even though 370 mg of sodium is only 15 per-cent of the Daily Value, by eating an entire bag you've tripled that and consumed 1,110 mg—nearly half the amount (2,400 mg) recommended by the American Heart Association.

**CONSUMER ALERT** Pregnant women; anyone with high blood pressure, gastrointestinal problems, or cardiovascular concerns.

**No Artificial Flavors** Products so labeled can still contain "natural fla-vors," which are chemicals that occur in nature and may contain sub-stances such as MSG (monosodium glutamate) and HVP (hydrolyzed vegetable protein) to which many people are sensitive. (See section 28.) Products that contain "natural flavors" usually indicate that the real thing (usually fruit) is left out. Ironically, "natural flavors" appear most often in junk foods.

**CONSUMER ALERT** Allergic individuals, pregnant and lactating women, hyperactive children.

**Reduced Calorie** This describes a nutritionally altered product with at least 25 percent fewer calories per serving than the regular or reference food. Be aware, though, that reduced-calorie food may contain more than you want of artificial sweeteners or sodium.

**CONSUMER ALERT** Dieters, allergic individuals, people with high blood pressure or gastrointestinal concerns.

**No Preservatives** Products that boast "no preservatives" can still con-tain them (they can be in the ingredients the manufacturer buys to make the products), as well as artificial colors and other additives.

**CONSUMER ALERT** Allergic individuals, women who are pregnant or breast-feeding, hyperactive children.

**No Cholesterol** This is frequently used to make a product seem more nutritious—and worth paying more for—but is virtually meaningless when used on foods from plant sources such as peanut butter or margarine, since the only foods with cholesterol are of animal origin. No cholesterol does *not* mean no fat! (Cholesterol is just one type of fat.)

**CONSUMER ALERT** Cost-conscious shoppers, dieters, anyone with cardiovascular problems.

**Cholesterol Free**    Just because it's "free" doesn't mean it isn't there. Products claiming to be cholesterol free have less than 2 mg of cholesterol per serving, and 2 g or less of saturated fat per serving.

**CONSUMER ALERT** Anyone with cardiovascular problems.

**Saturated Fat Free**    Once again, be aware that "free" isn't a guarantee that the product contains no saturated fat. All that it does guarantee is that there are less than 0.5 g of saturated fat and 0.5 g of trans-fatty acids in a serving.

**CONSUMER ALERT** Anyone with cardiovascular problems, dieters.

**Natural or All Natural**    When used on a meat or poultry label, "natural" means that the product doesn't contain any artificial ingredients or chemical preservatives. (This, regrettably, does not mean that the animal, when alive, wasn't fed artificial ingredients or chemicals.) On other products, the term *natural* may refer to specific ingredients and is therefore no guarantee that the product itself is free of additives or that it does not contain genetically modified ingredients.

**CONSUMER ALERT** Allergic individuals, women who are pregnant or breast-feeding, hyperactive children.

**Naturally Sweetened**    Once again, since "natural" has no legal FDA definition, calling a product "naturally sweetened" means little except for increasing sales. Be it honey, brown sugar, or corn syrup, a "naturally sweetened" product is neither necessarily lower in calories nor better for your health.

**CONSUMER ALERT** Dieters, children.

**Sodium Free**   This does not mean the product is *free* of sodium, only that a serving has less than 5 mg.

**CONSUMER ALERT**  Anyone with high blood pressure or cardiovascular problems, pregnant women.

**Unsalted, Salt Free, and No Salt Added**   Though no salt was added during the processing, "unsalted," "salt free," and "no salt added" products can still contain sodium—and depending on how much, or how often, you eat these products, you're probably getting more than you want in your diet.

**CONSUMER ALERT**  Anyone with high blood pressure or cardiovascular problems, pregnant women.

**Sugarless**   This means free of sugar (sucrose), but not necessarily free of other sweeteners (see section 80), and therefore sugarless products can contain just as many calories as those with sugar. If so, the fine print must state this, or something to the effect that the product is not dietetic but does not promote tooth decay. Regrettably, not many consumers take the time to read the fine print.

**CONSUMER ALERT**  Dieters, anyone with gastrointestinal problems (mannitol and sorbitol can cause cramps, gas, bloating, and diarrhea).

**Sugar Free**   Free can be costly if you overindulge in "sugar-free" products. Although by law there are less than 0.5 g of sugar per serving, serving sizes for different sugar-free products vary—as do people's appetites for them. And generally, these products contain artificial sweeteners.

**CONSUMER ALERT**  Dieters, anyone with gastrointestinal problems, children with allergies.

**Wheat Bread, Crackers, or Cereal**   Manufacturers can present an image of whole wheat by calling a product "natural wheat" or "stone ground wheat," but unless "whole wheat" is first on the ingredient list you're not getting the whole truth—or whole wheat.

**CONSUMER ALERT**  Diabetics, dieters, anyone with gastrointestinal problems.

## 8. Label Highs and Lows at a Glance

The term *high* can be used if the food contains 20 percent more of the Daily Value for a particular nutrient in a serving than the regular product.

The term *low* can be used on foods that can be eaten frequently without exceeding dietary guidelines for fat, saturated fat, cholesterol, sodium, and calories.

- **High fiber:** Must have 5 g or more of fiber per serving.
- **Low fat:** 3 g or less of fat per serving.
- **Less fat:** 25 percent or less fat than the comparison food.
- **Low calorie:** 40 calories or less per serving.
- **Low cholesterol:** 20 mg or less of cholesterol per serving and 2 g or less saturated fat per serving.
- **Low sodium:** 140 mg or less per serving.
- **Very low sodium:** 35 mg or less per serving.

## 9. How Fresh Is "Fresh"?

Although not mandated by the NLEA, the FDA has issued regulations for the term *fresh*. When it is used to suggest that a particular food is raw or unprocessed, "fresh" can be used only on a food that is raw, has never been frozen or heated, and contains no preservatives. That makes sense; but *irradiation at low levels is allowed!*

"Fresh frozen," "frozen fresh," and "freshly frozen" can be used for foods that are quickly frozen while still fresh. Still, *blanching (quick scalding before freezing to prevent nutrient breakdown) is allowed.*

## 10. What Manufacturers Can Say and What They Mean

If a product label boasts the claim . . .

- **"Healthy":** The food must be low in fat, saturated fat, cholesterol, and sodium, and contain at least 10 percent of the Daily Values for vitamin A, vitamin C, iron, calcium, protein, or fiber.

UNSAFE AT ANY MEAL

- **"More":** A serving of that product, whether altered or not, contains a nutrient that is at least 10 percent of the Daily Value more than the reference food.
- **"Fortified," "enriched," "added," "extra," "plus":** A serving of products making these claims must contain a nutrient that is at least 10 percent of the Daily Value more than the reference food—and in these cases the food *must* be altered.
- **"Rich in" or "excellent source":** The food contains 20 percent or more of the Daily Value for a particular nutrient in a serving.
- **"Good source of" or "added":** A serving of the food provides 10 percent more of the Daily Value for a given nutrient than the reference food.
- **"Little," "few," or "low source of":** Contains an amount that would allow frequent consumption of the food without exceeding the Daily Value for the nutrient. The product may only make this claim, however, as it applies to all similar foods.
- **"Fewer," "reduced," or "less":** The product contains at least 25 percent less of a given nutrient or calories than the reference food.

**COMMENTS AND CAUTIONS**  A "nondairy" product can still contain milk proteins. *(When in doubt, call the manufacturer!)*


## 11. How Natural Is "Organic"?

The *organic* label is helpful in understanding what you're buying and how natural it really is, but only if you know what the term really means. The new regulations divide organic labeling into four categories.

- Products that are labeled "100 percent organic" must contain *only* organic ingredients.
- Products labeled simply "organic" must have at least 95 percent organic ingredients, by weight or fluid volume, excluding water and salt.

12

- Processed products that contain at least 70 percent organic ingredients may be labeled "made with organic ingredients," and as many as three of those ingredients may be listed on the front of the package.
- Processed products with less than 70 percent organic ingredients may list those ingredients on the information panel but may not carry the term *organic* anywhere on the front of the package.
- Products that are labeled "100 percent organic, "organic," and "made with organic ingredients" may display those terms and the percentage of organic content on the front of the package.
- A "USDA" seal may appear on products labeled "100 percent organic" and "organic"—but not on the two others.

**CONSUMER ALERT** Processed foods labeled "made with organic ingredients" may still contain chemicals and additives such as MSG. Read those labels carefully—and remember that the ingredients are in descending order of predominance. (If an "organic" wheat cereal doesn't have wheat as the first ingredient, you're being taken for a needless nutritional "joy ride.")

## 12. Check Those Serving Sizes

Although nutrition information on food labels is given per serving, consumers frequently overlook serving sizes, an oversight that can get any *body* into trouble.

Many a dieter has discovered this the hard way—by carefully counting calories and still putting on pounds. A 10½-ounce can of soup, for instance, might have only 70 calories per serving. But without checking the fine print for the manufacturer's serving size, *and* noting the servings per container (which are frequently more than you think), you're probably consuming almost double the number of calories you intended. Now, 20 calories more or less might not sound like much. But just five foods containing 20 unlisted calories, eaten on a daily basis, can make you 10 pounds heavier in a year. In ten years, that's 100 pounds!

Fortunately, serving sizes have evolved from the days when manufacturers could determine what size was best for them as opposed to what was best for you. Serving sizes are now more uniform—and must be listed in common household and metric measures.

The serving sizes on food labels are based on FDA-established lists of "Reference Amounts Customarily Consumed per Eating Occasion." ("Eating occasion" does not mean Thanksgiving or Christmas dinner!)

**CONSUMER ALERT** Items can qualify as one serving or two if they are more than 150 percent but less than 200 percent of the reference amount for that particular product. For example, the serving size reference for a can of soup is 245 g. This means that a 15-ounce (420 g) can of soup may, at the manufacturer's discretion, be labeled as either one or two servings—whichever makes it sound more appealing.

## 13. How to Find Hidden Ingredients

The important thing to remember when looking at an ingredient panel is that the list is in decreasing order of quantity. In other words, you get the most of what comes first and the least of what comes last.

Sounds simple, right? Wrong. As anyone who has ever read a label knows, it's not so easy to figure out what a product contains even when the ingredients are listed. Right now, at least one hundred sweet substances are identified as sugars in products on the market, and manufacturers rely on the fact that the average consumer cannot identify them.

Companies also count on consumers not being able to identify sodium, cholesterol, fats, and additives. But you can easily learn how, and the time to do it is now.

### SPOT THOSE SUGARS

- Ingredients on labels ending in "-ose" indicate the presence of sugar. (For example, fructose is fruit sugar; dextrose, chemically identical to glucose, is made from cornstarch; maltose is malt sugar, formed from starch by yeast action; lactose is the sugar in milk.)

- Honey, corn syrup, corn syrup solids, maple syrup, molasses, and cane syrup, among over a hundred others, are also sugars.

**CONSUMER ALERT** If you are on a ketogenic diet, and avoiding carbohydrates, also be on the lookout for ingredients ending in "-ol," such as mannitol, sorbitol, and xylitol, as well as sorghum and starch.

## SPOT THAT SALT

- Look for the words *salt* and *sodium* (either listed alone or in combinations such as sodium chloride, sodium stearoyl lactylate, sodium caseinate, and sodium citrate), and notice in what position (and how many times) they appear on the label.
- Watch for the chemical symbols Na and NaCl.
- Know that baking soda, baking powder, and MSG (monosodium glutamate) all spell "salt."
- Be aware that products containing shellfish (clams, lobster, shrimp) are naturally high in sodium. (See section 110 for sneaky high-salt foods.)

**CONSUMER ALERT** The Nutrition Facts label lists a Daily Value of 2,400 mg per day for sodium (the amount contained in 6 g of sodium chloride [salt]). Be aware that just 1 level teaspoon of salt provides about 2,300 mg of sodium.

## SPOT THAT SATURATED FAT

- If a label offers multiple-choice ingredients ("contains sunflower seed oil, coconut oil, and/or palm oil"), and one is an unsaturated fat (sunflower seed oil) and the other(s) saturated, you are probably getting more saturated fat than you think.
- Whole milk is a food with a whole lot of fat that a whole lot of people are not even aware of because they've never bothered to look at the label.

- Doughnuts and cakes, which most people just think of as sugar sources, can add a significant and potentially dangerous amount of fat to your diet.

**CONSUMER ALERT** If you're eating less than 2,000 calories a day, you're getting a larger percent of saturated fat per serving than listed on the label.

## 14. Foods That Don't Have to Tell

Not all foods have to be nutritionally labeled, and, regrettably, these are foods commonly consumed by some of the most vulnerable individuals in our society—seniors, children, and people who are ill.

Food served in hospital cafeterias does not need to bear a nutrition label. The government reasoning here is that cafeteria food falls in the category of "food served for immediate consumption" and therefore is exempt from labeling. The same is true for food served on airplanes, and that sold by food service vendors; for example, mall cookie counters, sidewalk vendors, and vending machines.

Deli, bakery, and candy store items are also exempt, believe it or not. This is because although these foods might not be for "immediate consumption," they are ready-to-eat products that have been prepared primarily on site.

Any food shipped in bulk, as long as it is not for sale in that form to consumers, is allowed to cross state lines nutritionally unlabeled.

Medical foods, such as those used to address the nutritional needs of patients with certain diseases, also require *no nutrition labels*!

Plain coffee and tea, some spices, and other foods that contain no significant amount of nutrients are also exempt.

Foods produced by small businesses may claim exemption, too, if their sales are less than a certain amount annually or if they have fewer than a certain number of employees.

## 15. Coping with Invisible Ingredients

When companies put labels on food they are responsible only for what *they* added to it. If they buy ingredients from manufacturers who have already presweetened, salted, or added additives to them, that need not be mentioned on the food label you see.

As for ingredients that have been genetically altered, see section 38 for a list of the primary suspects and the best way to spot them.

**YOUR BEST PROTECTION** Seek products with the least amounts of these ingredients, eat in moderation, and vary your diet. Remember that it is not necessarily *how much* sugar or salt or fat the food you eat contains but *how often* you eat foods containing them.

## 16. What's in a Flavor?

Let me put it this way: What you think you are tasting is probably not what you think you are tasting. If this sounds absurd, it's because it is. Natural flavors occur organically through the combining of many different natural chemicals. Once a flavor's basic composition is determined, laboratory scientists can concoct a facsimile "artificial flavoring" by isolating components from the natural source or synthesizing them chemically, and then adding whatever chemicals they want to create a more realistic (or economical) flavor.

Though the FDA is periodically informed of substances being used in flavorings, all a manufacturer has to do is declare (on the basis of minimal substantive testing) that a new artificial flavor is safe and it can be added to food without FDA approval or without listing the specific ingredients in the flavoring on the product label.

The frightening truth is that millions of us consume hundreds of flavorings daily—*and many of them have never even been tested for their potential to cause cancer, birth defects, or any other health hazards.*

## 17. Flavoring Labeling Translated

If a product does not actually *state* a flavor, such as "lemon" or "strawberry," or have a picture on the package that makes it look lemony or strawberryish, the manufacturer is allowed to list the ingredients as "natural flavors," "artificial flavors," or both.

This generalized and misleading information is unfair to all consumers and for some it is potentially dangerous. Undisclosed flavor ingredients may cause a variety of adverse reactions in sensitive individuals that might be mistakenly diagnosed and, if treated incorrectly, result in serious health complications.

**COMMENTS AND CAUTIONS** The FDA states "an artificial flavor is no less safe, no less nutritious, and not inherently less desirable than a natural flavor." In all cases? Not in my book!

## 18. Those Mysterious "Spices"

Have you ever wondered what those nameless "spices" on ingredient labels are? This is not surprising since they can be one or more of dozens that need not be listed because— by FDA designation—they are aromatic vegetable substances that season and have no nutritional value. If the spice adds color, as in the case of paprika, turmeric,

> **Just because spices occur naturally does not mean that they can't harm you.**

and saffron, it must either be listed by name or as "spice and coloring." Only garlic, onion, and celery seasoning, because they are considered food, must be specifically identified.

This sort of ambiguous labeling can be dangerous, especially for the more than thirty million Americans who are allergic to the tiniest amount of certain chemicals. Simply because most spices occur naturally, and relatively small amounts of them are used in a food, does not mean they can't harm you. Nor does long use ensure safety. Safrole, which comes from sassafras, was used to flavor root beer for years before it was discovered to cause liver cancer.

## 19. Are You Getting the Right USDA Grades?

The USDA is responsible for inspecting and grading meats, poultry, fresh fruits and vegetables, eggs, and most dairy products. The grading and quality marks are based essentially on little more than certain standards of cleanliness necessary for public health safety.

But as inadequate as USDA grading is, it can at least provide you with some indication of a food's quality. Also, by recognizing government marks, you're less likely to be fooled by private gradings, which are still used by many small businesses to disguise inferior meats and poultry.

## WHAT TO WATCH OUT FOR

*When buying fresh fruits and vegetables:* Be wary of crates without government stamps, such as "U.S. Grade No. 1," or that are not marked "Packed Under Continuous Inspection of the U.S. Department of Agriculture" or "Packed by [name of company] Under Continuous Federal-State Inspection." **BEST HEALTH BUY** Organic produce.

*When buying poultry:* Watch out for the lack of a state or federal inspection stamp (that is, "Inspected for Wholesomeness by U.S. Department of Agriculture P-42"), or a "USDA A Grade" stamp, which indicates quality. (Birds below "A" grade are often privately labeled "Premium" or "Quality" by store owners, so beware.) **BEST HEALTH BUY** Poultry that is certified "organic." This USDA-approved label means that the birds come from farms that have been inspected to verify that they meet standards mandating the use of organic feed, prohibiting the use of antibiotics, and requiring that animals have access to fresh air and sunlight.

*When buying meats:* Avoid any that are not stamped with the abbreviation "U.S. INSP'D & P'S'D." Meat that crosses state lines must be inspected for cleanliness. The mark is not on each cut, but should be on each carcass. (You can ask the store manager to show you the stamped carcass if you want to be sure you are buying safe meat.) Quality grading (for fat and marbling content; the highest is deemed "prime") is done at the packer's request, and each cut of meat is stamped ("Prime," "Choice," "Good," "Standard," or "Commercial"). Meats below "Choice" are not likely to sell well, so small markets will often supply their own grades, such as "Excellent" or "Top Quality." Canned, frozen, dried, or packaged meat products should have an inspection mark ("U.S. INSPECTED AND PASSED BY DEPARTMENT

OF AGRICULTURE EST. 38") to show that the food is sanitary and the label has been approved by the USDA for truthfulness. **BEST HEALTH BUY** Meat that is certified "organic." This USDA labeling means that the meat comes from farms that have been inspected to verify that they meet standards mandating the use of organic feed, prohibiting the use of antibiotics, and requiring that animals have access to fresh air and sunlight.

*When buying milk:* Avoid any that is not "Grade A" and pasteurized. Raw milk has more vitamin C than processed milk, but since milk is not a prime source of vitamin C, the risk of illness (cattle disease and tuberculosis can be transmitted to people through raw milk) outweighs its benefits. **BEST HEALTH BUY** Certified organic milk from grass-based dairies. Grass-fed cows have more omega-3 fatty acids in their milk than grain-fed cows.

## 20. Secrets of the Pyramid Revealed

The Food Guide Pyramid, which the USDA created to replace the old four basic food groups (fruits and vegetables, breads and cereals, milk, and meat), is designed to be used by all people, two years of age or older, and consists of five major food categories plus a miscellaneous one—which, sadly, is still far too often indulged in by far too many.

Taking the pyramid from the base up, where most of your selections should come from, here's the general guide for choosing a healthy diet:

**Breads, Cereals, Rice, & Pasta**  6 to 11 servings a day.
One serving = 1 slice of bread; ½ English muffin; ½ regular bagel;
    ½ cup cooked rice, pasta, or cereal; 1 oz. cold cereal.
**Vegetables**  3 to 5 servings a day.
One serving = ½ cup cooked or raw vegetables; 1 cup raw leafy vegetables; ½ cup vegetable juice.
**Fruits**  2 to 4 servings a day.
One serving = 1 medium apple, orange, banana, other fruit, or
    melon wedge; ¼ cup dried fruit; ¾ cup fruit juice.
**Milk, Yogurt, & Cheese**  2 to 3 servings a day.
One serving = 1 cup or 8 oz. of milk or yogurt; 1½ oz. natural
    cheese; 2 oz. processed cheese; 1 cup cottage cheese. (Choose

THE LOWDOWN ON LABELS

low-fat milk; low-fat or nonfat yogurt; and "part skim" or low-fat cheeses.)

**Meat, Poultry, Fish, Dry Beans, Eggs, & Nuts**  2 to 3 servings a day.

One serving = 2 to 3 oz. cooked lean meat, poultry, or fish (about the size of a deck of cards or the palm of your hand); 1 cup cooked legumes, such as black beans, pinto beans, kidney beans ("habicuelas"), split peas, or lentils; 2 eggs; 4 tablespoons peanut butter.

**Fats, Oils, & Sugar**  Use sparingly.

Butter, margarine, gravies, mayonnaise, alcoholic beverages, ice cream, cookies, chips, candies, high-calorie condiments, French fries. (All high-fat and high-sugar foods should be eaten only in moderation.)

## 21. Any Questions About Chapter 1?

*Does the "net" weight of a canned product mean the actual weight of the food without the liquid in which it's packed?*

The use of the word *net* might make it appear that way ("net income," after all, means what you actually have after deductions), but the answer is no. The net weight on labels means everything—water, syrup, and oil—that is contained along with the food in the can, jar, or package. The only thing deducted is the weight of the container.

One 6½-ounce can of tuna fish, for instance, might be more expensive than another brand, yet still contain less tuna.

*I'm very confused by the weights and measures used on most product labels. Do you have some sort of simple guide that can help an old shopper figure out how new foods measure up?*

The terminology is really less confusing than you think. The metric system is used for most RDI measurements of nutrients, and they are measured in very small amounts by weight—grams (g), milligrams (mg), and micrograms (mcg or ug).

For fat-soluble vitamins (A, E, D, and K) the system of measurement is international units (IU). IU measures the biological activity of a nutrient (its ability to support growth) rather than weight. Vitamin A values, though, are now also given in retinol equivalents (RE); that is, the equivalent weight of retinol (vitamin $A_1$, alcohol) *actually absorbed and converted.* Retinol equivalents come out to be about five to fifteen times less than international units. In the case of vitamin A, an RDA of 5,000 IU would be the same as 1,000 RE.

If that's more than you wanted to know, the following conversions should help:

## QUICKIE CONSUMER CONVERSIONS

1 kilogram = 1,000 grams (g) = 2.2 pounds (lb.)
1 pound = 16 ounces (oz.)
1 ounce = 28 grams = 2 tablespoons (tbsp.)
1 gram = 1,000 milligrams (mg)
1 milligram = 1,000 micrograms (mcg or ug)
1 gallon = 4 quarts
1 quart = 2 pints = 32 fluid ounces (fl. oz.)
1 pint = 2 cups
1 cup = 8 ounces
½ cup = 8 tablespoons (liquid) and 6 tablespoons (dry)

*How reliable are the current food labels for telling concerned consumers what we need to know?*

Labels on products from large companies are reliable in that they must meet government standards as specified in the sections above under penalty of law. But if you or your child is one of the six to seven million Americans with a food allergy, you can't always rely on even these labels. A recent FDA sample of baked goods, candy, and ice cream from more than eighty midwestern food companies found that products from a quarter of them surveyed contained allergens not mentioned on the labels—including peanuts, eggs, milk, and wheat. These allergens, it seems, frequently enter the product when baking sheets and utensils are reused.

Also, some labels, although accurate, are unclear. You should be aware that "casein," for instance, is a milk protein, that "semolina" indicates wheat, and that "albumin" is egg. The Food Allergy and Anaphylaxis Network suggests that allergic individuals always carry medicine with them, and be on the lookout for symptoms when young children eat unfamiliar foods.

## FOOD FOR THOUGHT

- The FDA recently examined eighty-five independent cookie and ice cream manufacturers and found nearly one-quarter of their products contained ingredients not listed.
- Half of the eleven members of the USDA advisory committee that helped establish the Food Pyramid—as well as federal food and nutrition programs—had ties to the meat, dairy, and egg industries, a fact that the USDA has kept secret from the public. The Washington, D.C.–based Physicians Committee for Responsible Medicine (PCRM) sued the USDA, late in 1999, charging that these meat, dairy, and egg interests would influence nutrition policy, and they won. PCRM cited, for example, that the guidelines promote dairy product consumption as a means of preventing osteoporosis—even though studies have shown that eating dairy products doesn't reduce the incidence of that disease. The lawsuit was, unfortunately, won too late to revise the current guidelines. In the future, though, the USDA will have to publicize the advisory committee selection.

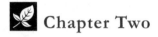 Chapter Two

# Those Unpronounceable Additives

## 22. What Additives Are

Additives are substances other than basic ingredients that are added to foods for numerous reasons, some of them praiseworthy, some appallingly not.

On the praiseworthy side, they are used to increase flavor, improve nutritional value, retard spoilage, extend shelf life, simplify preparation, and make more products readily available to consumers. On the negative side, they are used as adulterants to disguise inferior foods with dangerous dyes and chemicals so that manufacturers can make higher profits. (There are laws against this, of course, but they are difficult to enforce.)

An additive can be a naturally occurring food substance, such as vinegar (acetic acid), a chemical concoction such as BHA (butylated hydroxyanisole), or a combination of both (most artificial food flavors), but to qualify for use it must meet three FDA requirements:

- Perform a useful function in the food.
- Be safe for human consumption even if eaten in excessively large amounts over a lifetime.

- Not contribute to the growth of cancer in test animals, even when the amounts fed in laboratory tests are in excess of any amount possible for a human to consume in a lifetime.

Before any new additive may be used, it must be extensively tested for toxicity on animals. The only catch is that the manufacturer, not the FDA, does the testing.

## 23. Understanding the Myths

Considering that the average person consumes more than 4 pounds of food additives each year, it's unbelievable how little is understood by so many about so much.

### ADDITIVE MYTHS

- *All additives are bad.*
  All additives are not bad—at least not *all* bad. For instance, most preservatives used to prevent the growth of bacteria that cause deadly botulism offer benefits that outweigh their risks.
- *Some additives are completely safe.*
  No additive is completely safe for all people all of the time. The most innocuous additives—even ordinary foods, for that matter— are capable of causing adverse reactions during illness, for example, or if ingested while taking certain medications. Also, substances that are harmless for adults can be dangerous for children.
- *Foods in the old days were safer and more wholesome.*
  Foods have been adulterated for centuries. Two hundred years ago more dangerous additives were used than today. In fact, popular sugar confections contained mineral dyes that killed people every year.
- *Natural additives are safer than chemical ones.*
  Not necessarily. Coumarin, from tonka beans, was used for seventy-five years in flavorings before it was found to cause liver damage.

- *Naturally preserved meats are safe and chemical free.*
  Whether performed in old smokehouses or modern factories, the
  smoking process produces resinous, cancer-causing chemicals
  that are imparted to the food.

## 24. Unintentional Additives

Numerous manufacturing contaminants (detergents, solvents, lubricating
oils, textile fibers, plastics, and so forth) used in the production, storage,
and transportation of partially prepared foods or ingredients often wind
up in the final product. Because they weren't *intended* to be there, however,
they don't have to be mentioned on labels.

The same is true for antibiotics, hormones, and pesticides, the
residues of which not only can enter our foods, but also remain active
even after cooking and digestion.

This is particularly distressing since farmers use more than 2 billion
pounds of potentially carcinogenic pesticides annually, and only one hundred out of six hundred insecticide ingredients in use have been reviewed
for safety by the Environmental Protection Agency (EPA). Moreover,
only four of these have been completely tested for their toxic effects on
humans, and their long-term health hazards are still unknown.

## 25. The GRAS in Your Diet

Just because an additive has been declared GRAS (Generally Recognized As
Safe) doesn't mean that it can't harm you. When the food additive law requiring scientific testing of all chemicals for safe usage went into effect back in
1958, the FDA established the GRAS list to eliminate expensive testing of
what were unquestionably assumed to be safe chemicals (sugar, starch, salt,
baking soda, and so on). By doing this, all additives in use before 1958 were
deemed GRAS; unfortunately, quite a few were later found to be otherwise.

Though most of these have been removed from the list, many
of questionable safety remain, posing dangers that no one can afford
to ignore.

Think about these:

- GRAS additives have more liberal limits on concentrations at which they may be added to foods, and the foods to which they may be added.
- GRAS additives, unlike others, can be used by manufacturers *without prior FDA approval.* The FDA might later challenge such usage, but that is no consolation if your health has been irrevocably damaged.
- GRAS additives, because they are assumed to be harmless, are consumed in quantity and without question, and can therefore jeopardize the well-being of countless unwary individuals.

## 26. Some Popular GRAS Additives You Might Want to Keep Off Your Shopping List

### ACACIA GUM (Gum Arabic)

| | |
|---|---|
| Possible adverse effects | Mild to severe asthma attacks, rashes; has caused fatalities in pregnant animals. |
| High-risk individuals | Anyone prone to allergies, asthmatics, pregnant women. |
| Prime product sources | Soft and hard candies, frostings, gum. |

**MY ADVICE** There is a possibility that this additive may have mutagenic or teratogenic (abnormal embryo development) properties. If you're pregnant, trying to become pregnant, or a nursing mother, avoid products containing acacia or similar vegetable gums, particularly carrageenan (see section 87), gum tragacanth (fruit jellies, sherbets, and salad dressings), and carob or locust bean gum (flavorings for beverages, ice cream, baked goods, and gelatin desserts). See section 88 for safer trade-offs.

### ALGINIC ACID

| | |
|---|---|
| Possible adverse effects | Pregnancy complications, birth defects; has caused maternal and fetal deaths in animals. |

| High-risk individuals | Pregnant or lactating women. |
| Prime product sources | Ice cream, ice milk, fruit sherbet, frozen custards, cheese spreads, salad dressings. |

**MY ADVICE** Alginic acid (which is also used in the manufacture of textiles, artificial ivory, and glue) is still being investigated as a possible mutagen, capable of causing reproductive problems and birth defects. If you're pregnant, trying to conceive, or a nursing mother, limiting your intake of products containing this GRAS additive or other alginates (ammonium/calcium/potassium/sodium alginate; propylene glycol alginate; algin gum; algin derivatives) is highly recommended.

## BENZOIC ACID

| Possible adverse effects | Gastrointestinal irritation, asthma attacks, rashes, itching, irritation of eyes and mucous membranes, neurological disorders, hyperactivity in children. |
| High-risk individuals | Anyone prone to allergies, asthmatics, young children, people with liver problems. |
| Prime product sources | Jellies, jams, fruit juices, margarine, beer, pickles, bottled soft drinks, maraschino cherries, mincemeat, barbecue sauce. |

**MY ADVICE** Despite GRAS status, benzoic acid and its salt, sodium benzoate, have been implicated in causing hyperactivity in children and mild to severe reactions in allergic individuals; for dogs and cats, 2 g are lethal. Since this preservative combines with glycine in the liver, increasing that organ's workload, anyone with cirrhosis, hepatitis, or other liver ailments should consult a physician before consuming products containing benzoate additives.

## BHA (Butylated hydroxyanisole) and
## BHT (Butylated hydroxytoluene)

| | |
|---|---|
| Possible adverse effects | Elevated cholesterol levels, allergic reactions, liver damage, kidney damage, infertility, sterility, behavioral problems, loss of vitamin D, weakened immune system, increased susceptibility to cancer-causing substances. |
| High-risk individuals | Infants, young children, pregnant or lactating women, anyone with allergies or heart, liver, or kidney problems, asthmatics. |
| Prime product sources | Chewing gum, candy, instant potato flakes, breakfast cereals, gelatin, desserts, dry mixes for desserts and beverages, lard, shortenings, unsmoked dry sausage, freeze-dried meats. |

**MY ADVICE**  Both BHA and BHT have been found to affect liver and kidney functions. Though BHA has been shown to be less toxic than BHT, both are possible carcinogens, can cause allergic reactions, have potential mutagenic properties, and should be avoided by high-risk individuals whenever possible—and by everyone as much as possible.

## CAFFEINE

See section 56.

## IRON SALTS
## (Ferric pyrophosphate, ferric sodium pyrophosphate, ferrous lactate)

| | |
|---|---|
| Possible adverse effects | Gastrointestinal disturbances, tumors. |
| High-risk individuals | Anyone with hemochromatosis or ulcers, pregnant women. |

Prime product sources      Enriched bread, breakfast cereals, poultry stuffing, self-rising flours, farina, cornmeal.

**MY ADVICE** There has been limited and insufficient testing of the long-term and carcinogenic properties of these additives. There is no need for you or any member of your family to be a guinea pig; avoid these particular iron salts whenever possible.

## MSG
## (Monosodium glutamate, glutamic acid hydrochloride, monammonium, monopotassium)

Possible adverse effects      Allergic reactions (particularly burning sensations, facial and chest pressure, and headaches), eye inflammations, brain edema (excessive fluid retention), central nervous and vascular system problems.

High-risk individuals      Infants and young children, anyone with high blood pressure or other cardio-vascular problems, anyone with allergies (particularly to sugar beets, corn, or wheat), pregnant women.

Prime product sources      Chinese food, sodium-free salt substitutes, seasoning salts, soups, condiments, pork sausages.

**MY ADVICE** Glutamic acid and its salts are no longer being added to infant foods, as they shouldn't be. Foods containing glutamates should be avoided, or at least limited in their intake, by all children. Decreases in brain function and learning abilities have occurred in test animals. If you have an eye inflammation—or are preparing to have any eye surgery—keep glutamates out of your diet. Also, if you have high blood pressure, glutamic acids can weaken the protective blood–brain barrier, the membrane surrounding the brain, causing unwanted excitability. And since the placenta concentrates MSG, doubling the amount to which the fetus is exposed, it's wise for pregnant women to limit their intake.

## PROPYL GALLATE

| | |
|---|---|
| Possible adverse effects | Gastric irritation, asthmatic and allergic reactions, reproductive failures, liver and kidney damage. |
| High-risk individuals | Asthmatics, anyone with liver problems, children, anyone allergic to aspirin, pregnant women. |
| Prime product sources | Vegetable oils and shortenings, dry breakfast cereals, flavorings for beverages, snack foods, candies, gum, frozen dairy products. |

**MY ADVICE** Since propyl gallate is frequently used in combination with BHA and BHT, it can intensify the problems caused by those additives. Its potential carcinogenic and gene-altering properties have not been sufficiently tested, so I'd suggest waiting until they have been before ingesting large amounts of it. It has been banned from foods intended for babies and young children in England.

**CONSUMER ALERT** There are some other additives that you should be especially careful to avoid because they are either unsafe in the amounts in which they're consumed or have been very poorly tested. These are acesulfame K, potassium bromate (see section 53), saccharin (see section 80), sodium nitrate and sodium nitrite (see section 49), and sulfites (see sections 30–32).

## 27. Why Are Additives in My Food?

Additives have numerous functions, and almost as many terms and categories to explain them. The following are those most commonly seen, heard, and misunderstood.

## ACIDS

These are substances used frequently in many processed foods, particularly in breads and other baked goods to cause the desired "rising" (potassium acid tartrate, sodium aluminum phosphate, tartaric acid); in soft drinks to modify flavor (citric acid, malic acid, tartaric acid, phosphoric acid); in butter to help preserve flavor and retard spoilage (usually the same acids that are used in soft drinks).

## ALKALIES

These are used to neutralize excess acidity in such foods as cocoa products, candies, cookies, and crackers (ammonium hydroxide, ammonium carbonate).

## ANTIOXIDANTS

Antioxidants are preservatives for fats and oils to prevent rancidity and the development of off-flavors that can cause sickness. They are used in margarine, shortenings, lard, soup stocks, dehydrated potatoes, potato chips, salted peanuts, cheese spreads, and many more products (benzoic acid, BHA, BHT). Also, since oxygen activates enzymes that tend to discolor cut fruits and vegetables and make them less marketable, antioxidants such as sodium sulfite, ascorbic acid, and sulfur dioxide are used on these, too. (See section 30.)

## ANTISTALING AGENTS

These are used to prevent crystallization of starch, which makes bread turn stale, hard, and unmarketable. They are called bread emulsifiers but are actually antifirming agents (mono- and diglycerides, diacetyl tartaric acid esters of mono- and diglycerides, succinylated mono- and diglycerides).

## BLEACHING AND MATURING AGENTS

These agents improve the baking quality of flour by accelerating its oxidation while also functioning as yeast foods and dough conditioners

33

(potassium bromate, potassium iodate, calcium peroxide, ammonium or calcium sulfate salts, ammonium phosphates).

## BUFFERS

These are added to processed foods to control acidity or alkalinity (ammonium bicarbonate, calcium carbonate, potassium acid tartrate, sodium aluminum phosphate, tartaric acid).

## DOUGH CONDITIONERS

These are used in breads and baked goods to produce uniformity, despite variations in flour quality, by making dough drier and easier to work with (calcium stearyl-2-lactylate, sodium stearyl fumarate).

## EMULSIFIERS

Emulsifiers are widely used in margarines, shortenings, ice cream, baked goods, and many other processed foods to perform the previously impossible mixing—without separation—of water in oil (mono- and diglycerides, sorbitan monostearate), and oil in water (polysorbates, polyoxyethylene sorbitan fatty acid esters), to provide uniform smoothness and homogeneity. Lecithin, from egg yolks, is the most widely used natural emulsifier (it is in the federal Standards of Identity for mayonnaise), though lecithin from soybeans is being used more frequently in nonstandardized products.

## EXCIPIENTS

These are carrier substances for additives used in bread; a pharmacological term for any inactive substance used to bind an active one into a form for usage.

## EXTRACTS

Extracts result from passing alcohol or alcohol and water through natural essences, such as lemon, orange, banana, and vanilla. As flavoring solutions, they can be purchased in supermarkets for home use. Since they are often too weak for effective flavoring, their potency is allowed to be intensified by combining them with other natural flavors. The extract must contain at least 51 percent of the original fruit's flavor, however, to be labeled as its extract.

## FLAVOR ENHANCERS OR MODIFIERS

These are substances with virtually no flavor of their own that are used in soups, sauces, cheeses, and products containing meat, poultry, seafood, and other protein, to maximize flavor without having to increase the amount or quality of the product's ingredients (monosodium glutamate [MSG], see section 26). They are also used for intensifying flavor in chocolate, vanilla, and fruit-flavored foods and beverages, such as gelatin, desserts, soft drinks, and other high-carbohydrate products, as well as to mask the bitter aftertaste in diet foods and lower the sugar content of regular foods (maltol, ethyl maltol).

## HUMECTANTS

Humectants are moisture-control substances used to prevent foods, particularly icings, candy, and confections, from drying out (glycerine, propylene glycol, sorbitol) and to prevent table salt from caking (calcium silicate).

## LEAVENING AGENTS

These agents are used in bread and other bakery products to keep them light and obtain desired rising (mostly phosphates, such as monocalcium, dicalcium, sodium acid, and sodium aluminum phosphate, but also acids, described previously).

## NATURAL AND ARTIFICIAL COLORING

Contained in virtually all our processed foods in one form or the other (often both), color additives are used to keep foods looking the way consumers have been led to believe they should look—even if that is not the way they really *do* look. For example, some oranges are actually green (see section 47), but that's not the color we have been taught oranges ought to be, and few consumers would buy them that way. They would be even more reluctant to purchase foods that, without additive dyes, would discolor after processing and storage. Colorings can also make products appear to contain ingredients that, in fact, they don't. (For more on natural and specifically suspect artificial colorings, see section 86.)

## NATURAL AND ARTIFICIAL FLAVORINGS

All flavor additives are used to achieve long-lasting, uniform, consumer-preferred product tastes. They bring out desired flavors, conceal undesirable ones, and even create some (artificial bacon bits, for instance, which are made from soybean protein). Natural extracts, essential oils (highly concentrated flavors obtained from fruit rinds), spices, oleoresins (concentrated spice extracts), and combinations of synthetic and natural substances are used as flavor additives in hundreds of processed foods, particularly soft drinks, ice cream, baked goods, confections, syrups, margarines, and shortenings (ethyl acetate, propionate, maloneate, and butyrate; caproic acid; decylaldehyde; diacetyl).

## NEUTRALIZING AGENTS

These function the same way as buffers.

## POLYSORBATES

These are emulsifiers used to enhance the freezing qualities of ice cream and improve the texture of cake mixes (polyethylene 20, polysorbate 60, polysorbate 80).

## PRESERVATIVES

Preservatives retard the growth of microorganisms and help prevent spoilage and mold in virtually all processed foods. In bread, they are used primarily to extend shelf life and prevent mold (acetic acid, lactic acid, sodium and calcium propionate, sodium diacetate), as they are in cheeses, canned pie fillings, and syrups (sodium and potassium salts, sorbic acid). Because of their versatility, the most widely used preservatives are propyl gallate, sulfur dioxide, sugar, salt, and vinegar.

## PROPELLANTS

These are gases or easily vaporized liquids used as whipping agents for dessert toppings and to expel contents of other foods, such as processed cheeses and icings, that are sold in aerosol containers (nitrogen, carbon dioxide, nitrous oxide).

## SEQUESTRANTS

These preservatives prevent physical or chemical changes, caused by trace metals, that adversely affect the flavor, texture, or appearance of food, such as the premature setting of dessert mixes, discoloration of canned foods, and the clouding of soft drinks (EDTA [ethylenediaminetetraacetic acid] salts), as well as the loss of freshness and sweetness in dairy products (calcium, potassium, and sodium salts of citric, tartaric, and pyrophosphoric acids).

As sequestrants, EDTA salts are also used in beer to control the suds spritz that occurs when a can or bottle is opened.

## STABILIZERS AND TEXTURIZERS

These function much like emulsifiers, leavening agents, and thickeners. They keep ice cream consistently smooth and creamy by preventing water from freezing into grainy crystals. They also retard the settling of particles in liquid diet foods (eliminating the need to "shake well before using"), the cocoa particles in chocolate drinks, and the pulp particles in orange drinks, as well as improve the foaming properties of brewed beer (carrageenan, gelatin, carob bean gum, agar-agar, methylcellulose).

In cured meats, they are used to stabilize the pink color (sodium nitrate, sodium nitrite). (See section 49.)

## SURFACTANTS

These fall into numerous categories, such as emulsifiers, foaming agents, stabilizers, and more. They're used in peanut butter, for instance, to keep oil and water mixtures from separating; in salad dressings they're used as thickeners. (Cellulose derivatives and vegetable gums are often classified as surfactants.)

## SYNERGISTS

These are substances capable of increasing the effect of another substance. They are used to enhance the effects of antioxidant additives (citric and tartaric acid; calcium, potassium, and sodium salts).

## THICKENERS

Like stabilizers, emulsifiers, leavening agents, and other texturizers, thickeners are used to improve or maintain a product's desired body and consistency. They increase the firmness of canned tomatoes (amounts standardized by the FDA), potatoes, and sliced apples to prevent them from falling apart (calcium chloride, calcium citrate, mono- and dicalcium phosphate).

In artificially sweetened soft drinks, they're used to replace the body and thickness that would ordinarily be contributed by sugar. And in cheese spreads, gravies, icings, pie fillings, salad dressings, and syrups, they create any desired consistency (sodium alginate, pectins, natural vegetable gums which also work as stabilizers).

## 28. What They Can Do to You: Symptom–Additive Connections

Additive side effects are more common than most people (and many doctors) imagine, but they are usually assumed to be symptoms of other diseases—and treated as such. This is easy to understand, since Swiss cheese sandwiches for lunch would seem unlikely to be responsible for your migraines—but they could be! The same holds true for other discomforts, such as mouth or eye pains, which frequently send people off to dentists and ophthalmologists for medications they don't need.

Obviously, a doctor should always be consulted if any condition is causing consternation; but before rushing and getting a prescription (which is likely to have its own side effects), look over the following list and see if there is any relationship between the way you feel and the food additives you're eating; then be sure to discuss these with your doctor. *(This list is by no means all-inclusive, but it should give you a pretty good idea of the numerous symptom–additive connections there can be.)*

| SYMPTOM | POSSIBLE ADDITIVE CULPRIT |
|---|---|
| Anemia | Potassium nitrite |
| Asthma (breathing problems) | Acacia (gum arabic); acetal; allyl sulfide; benzoic acid; potassium nitrite; propyl gallate (all gallates); sodium nitrite; sodium, potassium, and calcium benzoate; sodium sulfite (and all other sulfites); tartrazine (or other azo or "coal tar" dyes |
| Blurred vision | Tartrazine (or other azo dyes) |
| Constipation | Aluminum hydroxide |
| Depression | Benzaldehyde; benzyl alcohol; butyl acetate |
| Diarrhea | Acetic acid; benzyl alcohol; calcium disodium EDTA; capsicum (cayenne pepper); L-ascorbic acid (vitamin C); mannitol; monopotassium glutamate; Olestra; potassium bromate; sorbitol; sorbitol syrup |
| Dizziness | MSG; sodium and other nitrites |
| Edema (retention of fluid) | Sodium acetate; synthetic "coal tar" or azo dyes |

| SYMPTOM | POSSIBLE ADDITIVE CULPRIT |
|---|---|
| Elevated blood sugar | Glycerol |
| Excessive thirst | Glycerol |
| Eye irritation | Acetic acid; biphenyl (diphenyl); butyl acetate; cornstarch |
| Faintness | MSG; potassium metabisulfite (potassium prosulfite) |
| Flatulence and bloating | Agar-agar; guar gum; pectin; sorbitol; sorbitol syrup |
| Flushing | Aluminum nicotinate; nicotinic acid (niacin nicotinamide) |
| Gastrointestinal upset or pain | Acetic acid; aloe extract; aluminum nicotinate; aluminum potassium sulfate; ammonium chloride; ammonium hydrogen carbonate; ammonium bicarbonate; benzoic acid; calcium chloride; calcium disodium EDTA; calcium gluconate; capsicum (cayenne pepper); guar gum; monopotassium glutamate; Olestra; polyoxyethylene stearates; potassium bromate; potassium chloride; potassium hydroxide; potassium nitrate; propyl gallate; sodium and potassium polyphosphates; sodium carbonate; sodium metabisulfite (and all sulfites); synthetic "coal tar" or azo dyes; tartaric acid |
| Hay fever | Cornstarch, tartrazine (or other azo dyes) |
| Headaches | Glycerol; MSG; sodium nitrite and other nitrites; sodium propionate |
| Heart problems | Acetal; calcium chloride; calcium gluconate; coconut oil; sodium carbonate; sodium sulfate |

| SYMPTOM | POSSIBLE ADDITIVE CULPRIT |
|---|---|
| High blood pressure | Acetal; indigo carmine (or other "coal tar" dyes); MSG |
| Inflamed or ulcerated colon | Carrageenan |
| Inflammation of the tongue | Caramel |
| Itching and hives | Cochineal or carmine; FD&C Blue No. 1 and 2 (or other "coal tar" azo dyes); MSG |
| Kidney problems | Aloe extract; allyl sulfide; ammonium chloride; bromated vegetable oils; EDTA; L-ascorbic acid (in large doses); magnesium sulfate (Epsom salts); polyoxyethylene stearates; potassium acetate; sodium sulfate |
| Liver problems | Allyl sulfide; ammonium chloride; propyl gallate (and all alkyl gallates) |
| Low blood pressure | FD&C Blue No. 1 and 2 (or other "coal tar" or azo dyes); MSG |
| Mouth ulcers or burning sensation in mouth | Aluminum, ammonium, or potassium sulfate; anethole; potassium hydroxide; tripotassium citrate (potassium citrate) |
| Nausea | Ammonium and potassium chloride; biphenyl (diphenyl); glycerol; guar gum; mannitol; monopotassium glutamate; MSG; sodium and other nitrites; synthetic "coal tar" or azo dyes |
| Nose irritation | Biphenyl (diphenyl); cornstarch |
| Overactive thyroid function | Erythrosine (a "coal tar" dye) |

| SYMPTOM | POSSIBLE ADDITIVE CULPRIT |
| --- | --- |
| Purple patches on skull | Tartrazine (or other azo dyes) |
| Raised cholesterol levels | BHA; BHT |
| Reproductive failure | BHT; cedar leaf oil |
| Scalp lesions, crusts, dandruff, hair loss | Caramel |
| Sensitivity to light | Angelica; bergamot; cedar leaf oil; clover; erythrosine (a "coal tar" dye) |
| Skin rashes | Acacia (gum arabic); acetic acid; alkyl sulfates; benzoic acid; benzoyl peroxide; cinnamon bark extract and oil; polyoxyethylene stearates; sodium, potassium, and calcium benzoate; sodium metabisulfite (and other sulfites); sorbic acid; tartrazine (or other azo or "coal tar" dyes) |
| Tooth or gum erosion | Citric acid |
| Urinary disorders | Ammonium chloride; EDTA; formic acid; sodium and calcium formate; polyoxyethylene stearates |
| Vomiting | Acetic acid; aluminum ammonium sulfate; ammonium and potassium chloride; benzyl alcohol; biphenyl (diphenyl); calcium disodium EDTA; chamomile; mannitol; monopotassium glutamate; potassium bromate; potassium hydroxide; sodium and other nitrites; synthetic "coal tar" or azo dyes |

## 29. The Silent Additive

It is called irradiation. You don't smell it; you don't taste it. But it's approved as an additive by the FDA and USDA, and is used on fresh fruits, vegetables, meat, poultry, wheat, shell eggs, herbs, spices, and dried vegetable seasonings—and *has not yet been proven conclusively safe for human consumption!*

Irradiation (a "cold sterilization" process involving gamma rays from nuclear material, x-rays, or high-energy electrons) has been used for many years to kill insects in wheat and flour and control microbial contamination of spices and seasonings, as well as to destroy parasites in meat and poultry—but not without taking its toll. By zapping food with ionizing radiation, free radicals *(bad guys),* uncontrolled oxidations that damage cells and weaken the immune system, are created. These free radicals frequently recombine to form stable compounds, some of which are known to be cancer causing (formaldehyde, benzene, lipid peroxides). Others have never been seen or studied before. These new compounds are called unique radiolytic products (URPs). Because scientists have not studied the long-term effects on humans of a diet of irradiated foods containing unknown amounts of URPs, *they cannot say that URPs have no health effects, or that a diet of irradiated food is safe!*

**IRRITATING FACTS ABOUT IRRADIATION**

- There have been no long-term human studies, and almost no studies on children to support safety.
- Food exposed to the same levels of radiation being used on poultry and meats for human consumption caused testicular tumors, kidney failure, death of offspring, and miscarriages in laboratory animals.
- Irradiation can damage vitamins A, C, E, K, $B_1$, $B_2$, $B_3$, and $B_6$ and folic acid up to 80 percent, depending on the vitamin and how long the foods are stored. *(And these are the vitamins most needed to fight the free radicals created by irradiation.)*
- All irradiated foods must be labeled using the "radura" symbol (a benign-looking flower within a broken circle) along with some

wording that the food has been specially processed—*but only to the first purchaser* (which may be a restaurant, school, or manufacturer), who is usually *not* the consumer.

- Irradiation labels are not required on foods prepared or served by restaurants, airlines, hospitals, schools, nursing homes, and other commercial establishments. They are also not required on deli or supermarket take-out foods, spices and herb teas, sprouts grown from irradiated seeds, ingredients in supplements, or plant-food ingredients that are processed again, such as apples in applesauce.

- Consumer labels on irradiated foods are required only for foods sold in their whole form (a *package* of chicken breasts, a *bag* of oranges, a *bag* of wheat flour); unpackaged meat and poultry (for example, from a butcher) is supposed to be labeled, too. On fresh whole vegetables and fruits, the notice is supposed to appear on a display card or on each single piece, but the requirement is often ignored and rarely enforced. By law, the notice must appear on multi-ingredient products that include irradiated meat or poultry (such as irradiated chicken in a TV dinner), but you have to look really carefully to spot it.

- Some foods may be irradiated twice, as in ground meat used in a prepared frozen chili that is also irradiated—but you, the consumer, will never know it.

- Fresh juices are now allowed to be processed with ultraviolet light—decreasing the vitamin C in orange juice by about 13 percent and damaging other vitamins.

- Healthy-sounding herb teas and supplement ingredients such as garlic can be irradiated without labels.

- Bacon was approved for irradiation in 1963. Five years later the approval was rescinded because animals fed irradiated bacon showed adverse health effects.

- Although organic foods cannot be irradiated, "natural" foods still can be.

- Fruits and vegetables irradiated up to the FDA maximum can be labeled as "fresh."

- Large food companies and irradiation advocates want the wording "treated with (or by) radiation" removed from consumer labels and replaced with something friendlier, like "electronically pasteurized."

**CONSUMER ALERT** Irradiation does *not* kill the prion that causes mad cow disease, nor can it kill viruses such as hepatitis or the Norwalk virus in shellfish. This can be especially dangerous because by eliminating telltale odors that indicate food has spoiled, that food may still contain bacteria and viruses that can cause life-threatening food poisoning.

## 30. The Sinister Six Sulfites

Sulfites have been removed from the GRAS list and banned from use on fresh produce and cut fruits and vegetables that are to be eaten raw, but there are still supermarkets, restaurants, and salad bars that continue to employ them. Sulfites function as sanitary agents (usually to compensate for unhygienic food processing practices) and preservatives to help prevent the discoloration of dehydrated, frozen, and fermented fruits and vegetables. They keep potatoes white and lettuce green, and they have been implicated in the deaths of at least thirteen persons.

Collectively they are known as sulfiting agents and go under the following names on ingredient listings:

- Potassium bisulfite
- Sodium bisulfite
- Sodium sulfite
- Potassium metabisulfite
- Sodium metabisulfite
- Sulfur dioxide

If you're asthmatic, prone to allergies, or deficient in the liver enzyme sulfite oxidase, they can kill you!

At present, these additives are banned from use on fresh fruits and vegetables (with the exception of precut or peeled potatoes that are used, for example, to make French fries or hash browns, and often potato salads in delis). Sulfites are also prohibited from being used on meat because they can restore red color and create a false appearance of freshness—but ingredients treated with sulfites may be added to meat in the preparation of processed foods, such as beef stew. (In this case the product label must include the specific name of the sulfiting agent or state that it contains "sulfiting agents.")

Sulfites, according to the FDA, are considered safe for *healthy* individuals who don't excessively consume foods or beverages in which they are present. The trouble is, they *are* excessively present. (See section 32.)

Reactions in sulfite-sensitive individuals can range from mild breathing difficulties to anaphylactic shock. Symptoms may include severe headaches, faintness, abdominal pains, nasal stuffiness, facial flushing, and diarrhea, either singly or in any possible combination. These reactions, unlike most allergic responses, occur quickly, usually within twenty minutes or so after ingestion of a sulfited food.

Sulfites also destroy vitamin $B_1$ (thiamine), which is why foods that are known to be major sources of this vitamin are not allowed to contain them. Yet, once again, a lot still do! For instance, many of today's bran cereals (fine thiamine sources) contain dried fruits preserved with sulfites. And though soy protein, canned vegetables, and fruit juices might not be *major* sources of thiamine, they are good ones, especially if consumed daily. Their sulfite content can negate any potentially significant vitamin $B_1$ contribution to your diet, however. Other nutrients depleted by sulfites are vitamin A (sulfites destroy 80 percent of the vitamin A in eggs), the B-complex vitamins, vitamin C, vitamin E, and beta-carotene.

## 31. Protecting Yourself Against Sulfites

If you have allergies, asthma, or suspect that you are sensitive to sulfites, you can protect yourself in several ways:

- Read labels and avoid foods with any sulfiting agents.
- If the food is being sold loose or by the portion, ask the store manager to check the ingredient list on the product's original packaging.
- Have your inhaler with you when you go out to eat. (If you've experienced a severe reaction to sulfites in the past, always carry

an antihistamine and an easily injectable epinephrine device, such as an EpiPen, to stabilize your condition until you get to an emergency room.)

- Avoid dried fruits. (Some asthmatics can have attacks simply from smelling a freshly opened package of dried apricots.)
- Don't have maraschino cherries in drinks or on desserts.
- If you want a potato with your meal, order a baked potato instead of fries, hash browns, or any dish that involves peeling the potato first.
- Throw away the outside leaves of any lettuce or celery purchased at supermarkets.
- Ask at restaurants if your food contains sulfites. (They might not know or they might not tell you, but it doesn't hurt to ask. If you're still worried, order something not sulfited—broiled chicken, meat, or an organic omelet without vegetables, for instance.)

**CONSUMER ALERT** There are sulfite strips sold at pharmacies that are designed to indicate the presence of sulfites by producing a virtually instantaneous red color when touched to a sulfite-containing food. But leading scientists in sulfite research at the Food Research Institute of the University of Wisconsin warn against the use of the strips unless users are carefully instructed in the procedures and are provided a list of foods that could give false positive or negative results. Inaccurate readings may be not only confusing but also dangerous.

## Mindell Vitamin Program

Taking nutritional supplements can help minimize allergic and asthmatic reactions. Here is my basic supplement regimen and foundation for general good health. An all-natural high-potency multiple vitamin and amino acid–chelated mineral complex (containing digestive enzymes for better absorption and no preservatives or artificial colors)

*and*

A broad-spectrum antioxidant formula (containing alpha- and beta-carotene, lutein, lycopene, vitamin C, vitamin E, selenium, ginkgo biloba, coenzyme Q10, bilberry, L-glutathione, soy isoflavones, grapeseed extract, and green tea extract)

Take each of these twice daily, A.M. and P.M., *with meals*. (Dosage is suitable for individuals over twelve years of age.)

**CAUTION** If you are on tetracycline medication, vitamin C buffered with calcium ascorbate can interfere with the medicine's effectiveness. You can use a sodium ascorbate form of vitamin C with tetracyclines, but *not* if you're on a sodium-restricted diet or are taking steroids. Check labels.

---

**IMPORTANT NOTE: Before starting any
supplement program—or making dietary changes—
you should check the cautions in section 142, pages 215–219,
and with your physician or a nutritionally oriented doctor.
*Regimens suggested in this book are not prescriptive
nor are they intended as medical advice.***

---

## 32. Know Your Most Frequently Sulfited Foods

Whether sulfites occur naturally, as they do in wines (without sulfites you'd have a lot of vintage vinegar), or are added later, they're equally dangerous if you have a sulfite sensitivity. Remember, just because a sulfite is not on the label doesn't mean it is not in the product.

### MOST FREQUENTLY SULFITED FOODS

### Baked Products

Cookies, crackers (even good old grahams), pie and quiche crusts, pizza crust, soft pretzels, waffles, flour tortillas

### Beverages
### (Canned, bottled, frozen, regular, and dietetic)

Beer, cider, cocktail mixes, colas, fruit drinks, fruit juices, instant tea, soups, vegetable juices, wine coolers, wines

## Candies, Confections, Desserts, and Syrups

Caramels, hard candies (sour balls and so on), brown sugar, raw beet sugar, powdered beet sugar, white granulated beet sugar, corn sugar, maraschino cherries, glazed fruits, jellies, jams, corn syrup, maple syrup, pancake syrup, fruit toppings, high-fructose corn syrup, shredded coconut, flavored (and unflavored) gelatins, fruit pie fillings

## Drugs

Antiemetics, cardiovascular drugs, antibiotics, tranquilizers, intravenous muscle relaxants, analgesics, anesthetics, steroids, and nebulized bronchodilator solutions (used for treatment of asthma)

## Fish
## (Frozen, canned, dried, and fresh)

Clams, crab, dried cod, lobster, scallops, shrimp; also canned seafood soups

## Pastas, Grains, and Other Carbohydrates

Spinach pasta, cornstarch, modified food starch, breading, noodle and rice mixes, potato chips, processed potato salad, hominy

## Relishes, Condiments, and Mixes

Horseradish, pickles, olives, onion relish, salad dressing mixes, wine vinegar, pickled vegetables, sauerkraut, coleslaw, guacamole, gravies (including those that are milk based), dried soup mixes

## Vegetables and Fruits
## (Canned, frozen, dried, instant, and bottled)

Mushrooms, grapes, prepared cut fruit or vegetable salads, shredded cabbage, avocado salad, dried fruits, trail mixes, breakfast cereals with dried fruit, dried fruit snacks, dietetic processed fruits

## 33. Vitamins Can Be Additives, Too

Vitamins are frequently added to foods for other than nutritional reasons and listed as ingredients under their chemical names. Since unfamiliar and unpronounceable ingredients have come to be regarded by health-conscious consumers as dangerous (admittedly, not without some reason), many nutritious products using vitamins as additives are being unnecessarily avoided.

A vitamin by any other name is still a vitamin—even when it's an additive. That doesn't mean vitamins are all risk free for everyone all the time (see section 142), but I believe their benefit–risk ratio as additives beats that of the competition's.

### VITAMINS AS ADDITIVES

| Vitamin | Possible Listing on Labels |
| --- | --- |
| A | Vitamin A acetate, vitamin A palmitate |
| $B_1$ | Thiamine hydrochloride, thiamine mononitrate |
| $B_2$ | Riboflavin, riboflavin-5-phosphate, sodium riboflavin phosphate (disodium riboflavin phosphate), lactoflavin |
| $B_5$ | Pantothenic acid, calcium pantothenate |
| $B_6$ | Pyridoxine hydrochloride |
| $B_{12}$ | Cyanocobalamin |
| $B_c$ | Folacin, folic acid |
| C | Ascorbic acid, sodium ascorbate |
| D | Vitamin $D_2$ (ergocalciferol); vitamin $D_3$ (cholecalciferol, 7-dehydrocholesterol) |
| E | Tocopherols, alpha-tocopherol, alpha-tocopherol acetate |
| G | Riboflavin (see $B_2$) |

H            Biotin, vitamin B factor

K            Menadione (vitamin $K_3$), menaquinone (vitamin $K_2$),
             phylloquinone (vitamin $K_1$), phytonadione

## 34. Any Questions About Chapter 2?

*Are there sulfites in dairy products?*

There are no sulfites in ordinary milk, butter, and yogurt, but they are in modified dairy products, such as filled milk, which is a specially prepared skim milk in which vegetable oils, rather than animal fats, are added to increase its fat content. Read your labels!

*I'm confused. Does a "fortified" product have more or fewer additives than an "enriched" one?*

Your confusion is understandable. Although fortification and enrichment are not the same, there is no legal distinction between them.

Essentially, fortification is adding nutrients to foods that never contained them (imitation fruit drinks, for instance). This means that inexpensive synthetic vitamins and minerals can be added to sugary junk foods to make them appear nutritious so they can sell for more.

Enrichment, on the other hand, is replacing nutrients in foods that once contained them. These nutrients are lost as a result of heat, storage, and so forth. Foods are enriched to the levels found in the natural product before processing.

Whether an enriched food has more additives than a fortified one depends on the product. My feeling, though, is to be wary of fortified products, since (with a few exceptions) most are just boosting their nutrient content to sell a naturally nonnutritious food for a greater amount of money.

*Could you please tell me what HVP is and if it's safe? And I would also like to know what it's doing in onion soup.*

Classified as an additive, HVP (hydrolyzed vegetable protein), sometimes called HPP (hydrolyzed plant protein), is frequently listed on labels as hydrolyzed cereal solids. (It's obtained through a chemical splitting of soybean and peanut meals, or crude protein from already wet-milled wheat, corn, or other grain by water-processing hydrolysis). I'd say avoid it as often as possible as it usually contains MSG (monosodium glutamate), which can cause allergic and other reactions (see section 26), and too much salt. Its prime use is as a flavor enhancer (frequently used in soup mixes, gravies, and chili to provide a meaty flavor), which is probably just what it's doing in your onion soup.

## FOOD FOR THOUGHT

- Oxygen-free packages can extend the marketable life of perishable foods from days to weeks or even months and deprive certain bacteria such as salmonella of the proper conditions for growth, but they encourage the growth of less common *Clostridium botulinum,* which can cause paralysis and death. They also give bacteria such as *Listeria monocytogenes* more time to multiply.
- Some food companies are trying to find a way to mask odors that result from increased shelf life. They're working on packaging that will trick consumers' noses into thinking the food they're eating is at the peak of freshness, by having the packages contain small flavors that burst when packaging is ripped open, releasing an appetizing aroma.

Chapter Three

# Genetically Modified Food Fright

### 35. What Are Genetically Modified Foods?

Genetically modified (GM) foods, also known as genetically engineered (GE) foods, are those that contain genetic material from another plant, animal, or bacteria, which changes the way they grow so they can battle bugs, fend off viruses, survive pesticides, and stay fresh longer.

Unlike nectarines (a peach and plum crossbreeding) or tangelos (tangerines crossed with grapefruits), which were foods crossed with related genes, today's genetic engineers transfer genes between *totally unrelated living things* to produce combinations that would never occur naturally, like fish and strawberries, viruses and vegetables—and the FDA still does not require mandatory labeling of all bioengineered ingredients or special safety testing before these products reach consumers!

### 36. Biotech Terms to Come to Terms With

GM: Genetically modified
GMOs: Genetically modified organisms

GE: Genetically engineered or genetic engineering

GEOs: Genetically engineered organisms

*Roundup Ready:* This describes genetically altered crops (namely, soybeans and corn) that contain a bacterium gene that makes them immune to the herbicide Roundup, enabling farmers to increase their production and profits by spraying without killing the crops. More than 90 percent of U.S. cotton is genetically altered. The popular varieties of biotech cotton are either immune to Roundup or produce their own pesticide. Most biotech corn being planted today makes its own pesticide.

*Bt* (Bacillus thuringiensis): This is a bacterial insecticide that is plugged into the genes of corn, potatoes, and cotton, after which the plants produce the insecticide themselves.

> **In the United States, two-thirds of our processed food contains genetically modified ingredients, and most people don't even know it.**

## 37. Gee, GE Is Risky Business

How risky are GE foods? Well, chew on these tidbits:

- Antibiotic-resistant genes are incorporated into nearly every GE organism. This could lead to the creation of a superbacteria, undermining the effectiveness of antibiotics as medicines, and lead to the development of new, antibiotic-resistant strains of bacteria causing infectious and life-threatening diseases.
- Genetic engineering can damage or alter the functioning of the natural genes in an organism and cause unanticipated toxins, allergens, and reduced nutritional content in foods. (Roundup Ready soybeans, which make up half of the soybean crop in the United States, have shown as much as a 20 percent drop in valuable phytoestrogens, beneficial in fighting osteoporosis and heart disease.)

- If genes from another organism are inserted into a plant, consumers will no longer be able to recognize allergy-causing foods.
- The prevalence of pesticides in the environment and the food chain exposes our ecosystem to irreversible pollution.
- There is no way to know for certain what the long-term effect of GE foods will have on humans or the environment.

> "Scientists found that putting sixty genetically engineered fish into a population of 60,000 native fish could render the entire species extinct in as little as forty years."
> —Joseph Mendelson, J.D., Legal Director, Center for Food Safety

- Bt crops, where the Bt gene has been engineered into the DNA of the food, continually produce toxins inside every cell of the vegetable all the time. The EPA registers Bt crops as pesticides, not vegetables—and they don't have to be labeled!
- Acres of crops with an unnatural genetic uniformity could be totally destroyed if a new fungus, bacteria, or virus adapts to them.

## 38. How to Spot the Usual Unusual Suspects

If you buy processed foods and want to avoid genetically engineered ingredients, suspect all that are listed below. If the label doesn't explicitly qualify them as "organic," you are probably eating more from the chemical crockpot of GM products than you realize.

- SOYBEANS (SOY FLOUR, SOY OIL, LECITHIN, SOY PROTEIN ISOLATES AND CONCENTRATES)
  **Products Prone to Containing Them**
  Popcorn, peanut butter, tofu dogs, cereals, veggie burgers, tamari, soy sauce, chips, ice cream, frozen yogurt, infant formula, sauces, protein powder, margarine, soy cheeses, crackers, breads, cookies, chocolates, candies, fried foods, enriched flours and pastas, nonorganic dried fruits

- CORN (CORN FLOUR, CORN STARCH, CORN OIL, CORN SWEETEN-
  ERS, CORN SYRUPS)
  **Products Prone to Containing Them**
  Tortilla chips, candies, popcorn, ice cream, salad dressings,
  tomato sauces, breads, cookies, cereals, baking powder, alcohol,
  vanilla, pie fillings, margarine, soy sauce, fried foods, powdered
  sugar, enriched flours and pastas
- POTATOES (POTATO STARCH, POTATO FLOUR)
  **Products Prone to Containing Them**
  French fries, instant mashed potatoes, restaurant potatoes served
  mashed or home fried, potato chips, Passover products that use
  potato flour, vegetable soups, vegetable pot pies
- COTTON (COTTONSEED OILS)
  **Products Prone to Containing Them**
  Processed food, peanut butter, potato chips, crackers, cookies
- CANOLA (CANOLA OILS)
  **Products Prone to Containing Them**
  Salad dressings, cookies, margarine, soy cheeses, fried foods
- PAPAYAS
  **Products Prone to Containing Them**
  Fruit salads, fruit drinks
- SQUASH
  **Products Prone to Containing Them**
  Vegetable stews, vegetable pot pies
- BEETS (SUGAR BEETS)
  **Products Prone to Containing Them**
  Horseradish, vegetable chips, candies, processed foods
- TOMATOES
  **Products Prone to Containing Them**
  Canned tomato products, pizza, vegetable soups

**COMMENTS AND CAUTIONS** Be aware that virtually all commercial yeast is
produced using some form of genetic modification. (Beer drinkers now
have something else to worry about. See section 91.)

## 39. Who Can You Trust?

According to Greenpeace's True Food Network's GMO facts (www.true-foodnow.org) at the time of this writing, these are some of the companies that do *not* use genetically modified ingredients.

| | |
|---|---|
| Amy's Kitchen | Gardenburger |
| Annie's Naturals | Gerber (baby foods) |
| Arrowhead Mills | Haine/Celestial |
| Balance Bars | H.J. Heinz Company (baby foods) |
| Barbara's Bakery | Mad River Sodas |
| Bearitos | Nature's Path Foods |
| Ben & Jerry's | Newman's Own |
| Birds Eye | Stonyfield Farm |
| Down to Earth | Wild Oats Drinks |
| Eden Foods | Yves Veggie Cuisine |
| Earth's Best (baby foods) | 365 Brand Whole Foods |
| Freshlike | |

**COMMENTS AND CAUTIONS** Shop organic, minimize your intake of processed foods, and reduce visits to fast-food restaurants. When in doubt, contact the manufacturer and ask for confirmation that its product contains no genetically modified ingredients, or ingredients derived from GMOs.

## 40. Genetically Unmodified Facts

- The only testing of genetically engineered food in the United States is on rats, by the genetic engineering companies themselves—a process that's only preliminary with food additives and pharmaceuticals.
- Aside from the issues of killing involved in the production of plant/animal combinations, most GM companies still test their herbicide and pesticide poisons on animals, causing unnecessary suffering and death.
- Genetic engineering totally ignores vegetarians and people with religious, cultural, or ethical strictures about animal

contamination of their food. Unlabeled GMOs for these people are morally reprehensible.

- Scientists at the Institute of Virology in Oxford, England, have introduced the gene responsible for scorpion poison into a potato as a pesticide.
- Half of monarch butterfly caterpillars that ate milkweed dusted with pollen from corn containing Bt died after four days.
- In the 1980s, to accelerate production of the amino acid food supplement tryptophan, the company Showa Denko K.K. added genetically engineered bacteria to its product and put it on the market. Within a few months, it caused the deaths of thirty-seven people and caused 1,500 more to become permanently disabled.
- StarLink corn, which contained the Bt herbicide gene, had a higher amount of toxin in its tissues and was approved by the EPA for use as animal feed. (Looking back, the EPA now concedes it should have been denied for animals and people equally.) But either by mechanical means or human error, it got into our food supply in the fall of 2000, causing hundreds of recalls, starting with Kraft's Taco Bell taco shells, and innumerable allergic reactions. Aventis, the manufacturer of StarLink, claims that the amounts of the protein found in the consumer foods was too low to induce allergic responses, to which Rebecca Goldburg, senior scientist at Environmental Defense replied in the *Wall Street Journal*, "There is no way a credible scientist could rule out CRY9C as a potential human allergen. I'm especially concerned about the risk to children, who are much more vulnerable to allergies than adults."

## 41. The Functions of Functional Foods

Functional foods are foods that claim to provide a specific health benefit above and beyond their inherent nutritional value. Some of these are foods containing naturally occurring substances that provide health benefits (cranberry juice, for instance, contains an antiadhesion component that may help prevent urinary tract infections), while others (such as Benecol, a margarine created to lower cholesterol) are designed by manufacturers with specific health benefits in mind.

Functional foods either contain additives that, according to the manufacturers, give them totally new nutritional qualities, or they have had certain qualities eliminated (such as allergens), thereby making them appear healthier.

**COMMENTS AND CAUTIONS** Even if an ingredient in food is healthy, you can still have too much of it. Adding vitamins may be beneficial to a person suffering from a deficiency but could be detrimental to someone else. An oversupply of vitamin $B_1$ (thiamin), for instance, can affect thyroid and insulin production.

## 42. Foodraceuticals

### A SAMPLING OF MANUFACTURED ONES

*Benecol:* A margarine-type spread that contains pine tree by-products, blocking the absorption of cholesterol in the intestine. It lowers LDL (bad) cholesterol, doesn't affect HDL (good) cholesterol, and is available as Benecol Regular (45 calories and 5 grams of fat per serving) and Benecol Light (30 calories and 3 grams of fat per serving). Three servings of 1½ teaspoons a day has been shown to reduce LDL by up to 14 percent within a few months. (Benecol also comes as a salad dressing and a snack bar.)

*Take Control:* Similar to Benecol, Take Control is a margarine-type spread made from soybean extracts, blocking the absorption of cholesterol in the intestine. Take Control (50 calories, 6 g of fat per serving) comes in tubs or packages of 1-tablespoon portions. Using 1 to 2 tablespoons a day has been shown to reduce cholesterol by an average of 7 to 10 percent.

**CONSUMER ALERT** Though you have to consume Take Control less often than Benecol, a tablespoon is a lot on a piece of toast. According to the National Association of Margarine Manufacturers, Americans consume less than 2 teaspoons of margarine a day.

*BetaSweet:* A maroon carrot bred to contain increased amounts of beta-carotene and anthocyanin, natural antiaging and anticancer compounds.

*Coming soon to a supermarket near you:* A potato that will absorb less oil during processing, resulting in lower-fat French fries and chips; non–GM soybeans with lower levels of trans-fatty acids; vaccines bred into bananas to combat common diseases such as hepatitis B; and rice with higher zinc, iron, and vitamin levels.

## A MARKET BASKET OF NATURE'S NATURALS

*Apples:* Good source of pectin, a soluble fiber found to reduce cholesterol, which can help to prevent heart disease.

*Bananas:* A natural antacid that quells the fires of heartburn; a great source of potassium which helps maintain normal fluid and electrolyte balance. A practically perfect food.

*Blueberries:* High in pectin, which can help lower cholesterol, blueberries contain antioxidants which may help prevent different forms of cancer as well as increase resistance to infections.

*Cranberry juice:* Contains a component that has a "Teflon effect" on *E. coli* bacteria, preventing it from sticking to the endothelial cells of the urinary tract, which may help prevent urinary tract infections.

*Garlic:* Diallyl sulfide (DAS), a component of garlic oil, may deactivate carcinogens and help prevent the growth of cancerous tumors.

*Grapes:* Contain compounds which may counteract carcinogens and protect the cardiovascular system. (See section 95.)

*Mustard greens:* Cruciferous vegetables containing cancer-fighting compounds; rich in antioxidants.

*Oats:* Beta-glucan may reduce the risk of heart disease.

*Parsley:* A natural breath freshener.

*Soy:* High in fiber and rich in isoflavones. In the body isoflavones are converted into phytoestrogens (plant estrogens) that may help block the growth of hormone-dependent and other cancers, and also may lower LDL cholesterol and protect against heart disease.

*Spinach:* Rich in folic acid (which helps prevent birth defects), beta-carotene, and iron.

*Yogurt:* Added lactobacillus culture may improve digestion.

## 43. Misfunctional Foods

One of the largest areas of expansion in the food industry is spiking foods with ingredients to enhance their healthful properties. But the claims being made for some of these foods have come under fire from the Center for Science in the Public Interest (CSPI). In fact, it has urged the FDA to halt the sale of dozens of these functional foods that contain ingredients not considered by the agency to be safe and because of false claims about the products.

Among the products named for their "Hall of Shame":

- Snapple's "Moon" Tea Drink, which contains kava kava. It claims to "enlighten your senses." Unfortunately, kava kava has been a factor in several arrests for driving while intoxicated. Kava kava is also used in Apple & Eve's Tribal Tonics' "Relaxation Cocktail" and Hansen's "d-stress" sparkling drink.

**COMMENTS AND CAUTIONS** Kava kava, a plant grown in the Polynesian and South Sea Islands, has slight hypnotic properties, and has been known to produce a mild euphoria. Long-term use of the herb can cause liver damage.

- Ben & Jerry's "Tropic of Mango Smoothie," which contains echinacea, and can cause allergic reactions—including asthma attacks in susceptible individuals—and can counteract drugs that suppress the immune system.
- Arizona's "Rx Memory Elixir," which contains ginkgo biloba, and is labeled as "mind enhancing." Ginkgo biloba can be a blood thinner in large dosage and can counteract anticoagulant drugs and increase the risk of excessive bleeding or stroke.

**COMMENTS AND CAUTIONS** Although the herb itself has been known to aid in mental functioning, it should only be taken as a standardized herbal extract. Taking it with aspirin may result in bloodshot eyes.

- Procter & Gamble's "Spire Energy with VitaLift Green Tea and Juice Beverage," which contains guarana extract. The label claims it provides "smooth, steady, sustained energy." The FDA has stated that guarana is not considered a safe ingredient for use in food.

**COMMENTS AND CAUTIONS** The seeds of the guarana plant contain up to 5 percent caffeine. The amount in the extract would be even more concentrated. Excessive intake of methylxanthines, a group of compounds to which caffeine belongs, has been linked to fibrocystic breast disease and prostate problems.

## 44. Any Questions About Chapter 3?

*Are functional foods all genetically modified?*

Not as yet. Most of the functional food on the market today is processed food, where the extra "function" is added during the processing, and not through genetic manipulation.

*I don't understand all the objections to genetically engineered crops. I've read that they can alleviate malnutrition in Third World countries, and prevent vitamin-deficient kids from going blind. That's a good thing.*

That would be a good thing, if it were true. The corporations that are manufacturing these crops are in it for the money. They're not going to *give* their products away. And even if people in these countries could afford the crops, they might have to depend on the corporations to provide them with special fertilizers and pesticides in order to grow them locally. In other words, widespread adoption of GE crops could put control of the world's food supply in the hands of a few powerful organizations. And that is scary!

## FOOD FOR THOUGHT

- All that is required by the FDA to approve new genetically altered foods is for manufacturers to notify the agency 120 days before putting the product on the market and promise that it is "substantially equivalent" to a conventional counterpart. Labeling is purely voluntary.
- A study in 1998 showed that DNA from the genetically engineered food fed to pregnant mice ended up in their intestinal linings, white blood cells, and brain cells, as well as that of their fetuses. The same may happen with humans—and the long-term effects are totally unknown.

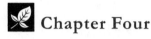 Chapter Four

# Is This Any Way to Start a Day?

## 45. The Meal Most Likely to . . .

Breakfast is the meal most likely to . . .

- Affect learning ability and reaction time.
- Influence vitality and fitness.
- Be rushed, unplanned, eaten on the run, and missed.

It is also the most important meal of the day—and the most nutritionally abused.

## 46. Breakfasts That *Don't* Make Your Day

Breakfast comes after the longest period of time that your body has been without food. If your internal systems are inadequately or improperly replenished, they are going to let you down. You can't expect high performance "running on empty."

Most people know this and feel that any breakfast is better than none. But you won't get high performance using the wrong fuel, either. Obviously, this is not as well known, as evidenced by the more than six million people who drink Coca-Cola for breakfast and the popularity of the following morning meals.

## THE OFFICE QUICKIE

This is a doughnut or pastry grabbed on the run and washed down with coffee. Regarded as a "something to hold you until lunch" meal, its subversive qualities, such as diminishing alertness throughout the morning and increasing midday fatigue, are not widely known—but they are experienced by millions daily.

*Trade-Off Suggestions:* Instead of a high-fat, high-sugar pastry, try a bagel. Bagels are low in fat, contain more protein than two slices of bread (with about the same amount of calories), and are now available with more fiber in whole-grain varieties. (A 3½-inch whole wheat bagel has 3 g of fiber, compared to the 1.5 g in a plain white bagel.) Instead of spreading it with cream cheese (which would defeat the trade-off since cream cheese has more than 2 teaspoons of fat per ounce), try tofu pâté, apple butter, or a really thin slice of Swiss or cheddar cheese topped with a tomato.

Low-fat cottage cheese mixed with either chopped scallions or fruit-flavored yogurt works well, too. But if you really feel that a bagel is not a bagel without cream cheese, use fat-free—or a *thin* layer of light cream cheese. You'll still have the flavor, but without all the fat, and be a whole lot healthier for it.

> **McDonald's Steak, Egg, and Cheese Bagel has 690 calories and 39 g of fat—and 14 of them are saturated!**

**CONSUMER ALERT** Bagels used to be about 3 inches in diameter and about 150 calories. Today, the average bagel is about 4¼ inches in diameter and has double the calories. And if it's an egg bagel, you're getting 35 mg of cholesterol, too! Size counts—a lot!

**CAUTION** Bagels are made with high-gluten flour and are contraindicated for anyone with celiac disease.

## FROZEN BREAKFAST SANDWICHES

Like Egg McMuffins (290 calories, 12 g of fat, 5 mg saturated fat, 790 mg sodium) and Croissan'wiches (510 calories, 36 g of fat, 14 g saturated fat, 1,530 mg sodium), microwavable breakfasts on buns are time-saving time bombs loaded with sodium and fat. One Swanson's Great Starts Breakfast Biscuit, for example, contains half your day's allotment for sodium plus a whopping 28 g of fat—with 11 of those grams saturated—and nearly 500 calories. Pillsbury's Toaster Scrambles are no better. This breakfast pastry, filled with real eggs, sausage, and cheese, has no fiber, and half its calories come from 12 real grams of fat. And as if this isn't bad enough, many of these breakfast products also contain additives (some potentially carcinogenic) that can cause numerous unpleasant reactions in susceptible individuals (see section 28.)

*Trade-Off Suggestions:* If you like the convenience of a hot breakfast on a muffin, but don't want all the sodium, fat, and additives that come with it, make your own. Spread an English muffin thinly with peanut butter, add a slice of low-fat cheese, microwave on high for about 40 seconds (or put in a toaster oven until the cheese melts), and you'll save a lot more than time. For variation, try low-fat cottage cheese, sprinkled with cinnamon, on a raisin muffin. Or, if you want more of a morning meal with less of a health risk, try my Way-to-Go Wrap. Just scramble up some Eggbeaters in a nonstick pan, stir in a cut-up, cooked vegetarian sausage, and wrap it all in a whole-wheat tortilla.

## NO-FUSS FRENCH TOAST, WAFFLES, AND PANCAKES

Now that they are microwavable, these classic breakfast treats are being served with increasing frequency in busy households, subjecting more unwary people, more often, to an unhealthy onslaught of excessive salt, sugar, potentially carcinogenic preservatives, and coal tar–based dyes. Though convenient and tasty, these no-fuss processed breakfasts can raise blood pressure, lower spirits, and, if eaten on a regular basis, become significant contributing factors to serious ailments.

*Trade-Off Suggestions:* If you're going to eat these breakfasts despite their nutritional negatives, compare the ingredients of different brands, then select whichever has the lowest amount of saturated fat and the highest amount of fiber. Choose products made with bran and whole-wheat flour over those that are not.

## FAST, FULL-COURSE FIRST MEALS

There is nothing like a good, nutritious breakfast—and the microwavable morning entrees now being marketed are nothing like good, nutritious breakfasts. Whether the meals sound down-home familiar (Great Starts Scrambled Eggs & Sausage with Hashed Brown Potatoes, for instance) or gourmet exotic (Cafe Classics Eggs Enchilada), the sodium and fat levels are equally and appallingly high. Cholesterol watchers, watch out! What these beat-the-clock breakfasts save you in time, you pay for in health. They contain between 360 and 500 mg of cholesterol—250 to 300 mg more than the amount recommended for a whole day!

*Trade-Off Suggestions:* If you want scrambled eggs and sausage, you're better off buying the sausage separately (choosing the brand with the least amount of harmful additives) and scrambling your own preservative-free, organic eggs. Also, heating up last night's leftovers can make a better full-course breakfast than you'll get in a box.

# 47. Getting the Juice on Juice

Frozen, canned, cartoned, bottled, or fresh orange juice is a real eye-opener—in ways that can make you think before you drink.

## JUICY EYE-OPENERS

- Orange juice is the most popular natural source of vitamin C, but not the best. (An 8-ounce cup of orange juice has approximately 124 mg of vitamin C; an 8-ounce cup of cooked broccoli contains 140 mg.)

- The vitamin C content of all oranges is not the same. (Different varieties contain different amounts, and these amounts increase or decrease depending on how early or late in their growing season the oranges are picked. Generally, the later they are picked, the lower their vitamin C content.)
- The vitamin C content of reconstituted frozen orange juice can vary from brand to brand by as much as 100 percent. (Wide variations in vitamin C content can also occur within a single brand.)
- All oranges are not orange. (Florida oranges are frequently green when they're ripe and dyed orange to please consumers.)
- The nutritional value of orange juice, fresh or processed, is highly overrated. (Except for its vitamin C and potassium, orange juice provides you with little more than carbohydrates in the form of the natural sugars sucrose, fructose, and glucose.)
- Fresh-squeezed or unsweetened orange juice is not a low-calorie drink. (It's actually higher in calories than many soft drinks.)
- A lot of expensive "fresh-squeezed" juice sold in cartons comes from last year's oranges. (As long as the oranges were fresh when they were squeezed, and the juice was not concentrated before it was frozen for storage, the manufacturer can blend last year's juice with current squeezings—squeezing out extra profits.)
- Canned and bottled juices (those that are stored and sold unrefrigerated) have about the same amount of vitamin C as frozen concentrates made from the same type of oranges being canned at a particular time, but their flavor tends to deteriorate. They also tend to have greater amounts of insect debris than other forms of orange juice. (Their only real advantage is that they can be stored without refrigeration. For ready-to-pour convenience, you're better off with reconstituted juice sold in cartons, which costs, ounce for ounce, about the same—with some store-label brand exceptions—and tastes better.)
- The FDA limits on amounts of "natural and unavoidable" debris in citrus juices are unappetizingly high, they don't cover all kinds of debris, and USDA inspection does not guarantee exceptional

cleanliness. (I'm not saying that allowable insect debris is a health hazard, but unless you're a bird, frog, or other arthropod eater by choice, it's certainly no taste advantage, either.)

- The good news is that as of January 18, 2001, makers of unpasteurized fruit and vegetable juices must follow strict steps—either pasteurization, treatment with ultraviolet light, or cleaning orange peels before squeezing the juice—to ensure their products aren't contaminated with salmonella or other germs.
- The bad news is that although the FDA inspectors will do spot-testing to make sure the system is working, there is no guarantee that they'll be able to spot the wrong spots at the right time.

**CONSUMER ALERT**  Many orange juice makers add concentrated scents to their containers before sealing them, so that when they're opened the juice smells really fresh.

## 48. Know Your Oranges

If you are going to squeeze your own juice, you're not likely to be helped in your selection by federal grade standards. Aside from the use of several grading systems (which is confusing when you discover that an orange grade "No. 1" is better than one graded "No. 1 Bright" as long as it is not from Florida, where that grade is reversed), oranges are graded primarily on appearance, shape, and color, which is not necessarily relevant to nutritional value or taste.

### DOs & DON'Ts FOR PICKING A GOOD JUICY ORANGE

DON'T buy any with soft spots, cuts, punctures, or spongy skin.
DO select the firmest and heaviest ones over the lightweights.
DON'T judge by color. (Many undyed oranges are greenish when ripest, and Florida and Texas oranges speckled with brown or black flecks are often thin skinned and top quality.)
DO choose those with smooth, fresh-looking skin.

DON'T select by name unless you know that variety's growing season. (Generally, the later in its season, the less the orange's vitamin C content.)

DO keep in mind that a medium-sized orange (approximately 6 ounces) will provide about 2 to 2½ ounces of juice. (The average small breakfast portion served is 3½ ounces.)

## GOOD NAMES, SEASONS, AND "Cs" TO REMEMBER

| Variety | Season | Approximate Vitamin C in 3½ Ounces of Juice |
|---|---|---|
| Valencia (CA) | April–October | 60 mg–42 mg |
| Valencia (FL) | Late March–June | 45 mg–22 mg |
| Temple (FL) | Early January–early March | 51 mg |
| Hamlin (FL) | Early October–December | 55 mg–36 mg |
| Pineapple (FL) | December–February | 60 mg–50 mg |
| Parson Brown (FL) | Early November–January | 52 mg–47 mg |

## 49. Hold the Bacon, Please!

There is nothing bad about bacon that not eating it won't cure. It's high in saturated fat and high in sodium. It contains nitrite, an additive that can react with natural chemicals in our foods and bodies to form nitrosamines, potent cancer-causing substances. And to heighten the health risks, it is an inconsistent product at best.

A pig's age, gender, and diet affect how it accumulates fat. This causes significant variations in the pork bellies manufacturers buy for use as bacon. Consequently,

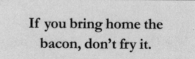

**If you bring home the bacon, don't fry it.**

taste, as well as protein, fat, sodium, and so forth, can vary not only from brand to brand but from package to package!

But more than quality and uniformity are involved. Even though there are legal limits to the amount of nitrites allowed, and specified vitamin C compounds that must be added to retard nitrosamine formation during processing, the product's inconsistency precludes assurance that every package of bacon has nitrosamine levels within USDA standards. In other words, the chances of your bacon having more nitrosamines than it should are more than likely. Add to that the fact that no level of nitrosamine is "safe," and you have to concede that bringing home the bacon can be a health-risky business.

If you are a confirmed bacon lover, expecting you to give up your beloved morning breakfast treat because of its potential health hazard is as realistic as getting confirmed ("I-know-the-risks-and-I'm-still-taking-them") smokers to quit. But you can at least minimize the dangers to your health.

## CUTTING BACK ON BACON RISKS

- Select bacon with the most meat and least fat. (Nitrosamine levels are higher in fat.)
- Don't use bacon grease for cooking. (It contains nearly four times the nitrosamines as the bacon!)
- Instead of frying, cook bacon on paper towels in a microwave. (This produces less nitrosamines.) If you don't have a microwave, broil or oven-fry the bacon at a fairly low temperature. It will take longer, but fewer nitrosamines will be produced.
- Always cook bacon in a well-ventilated area. (Some nitrosamines can vaporize during cooking, and they are easily inhaled.) It's wise to discourage young children in particular from sniffing those cooking aromas.
- Use nitrite-free bacon. (It's not as tasty, but it's not as dangerous, either.)

- Don't be fooled into thinking that baconlike products (Sizzlean, Tastystrips, and so on) are safer than the real thing. They use sodium nitrite for their cured taste and pink/red color, too.
- Eat bacon as an occasional treat. (Making it frequent or everyday fare is just asking for trouble.)

**MY SUGGESTION** If you do indulge in bacon, be sure you're ingesting enough vitamins C, A, D, and E to help counteract the nitrites. (For the best natural sources, see section 145.) I'd also recommend the following daily supplement regimen:

- An all-natural, high-potency multiple vitamin and amino acid–chelated mineral complex (containing no preservatives or artificial colors), preferably one with digestive enzymes for better absorption
- A broad-spectrum antioxidant formula (containing alpha- and beta-carotene, lutein, lycopene, vitamin C, vitamin E, selenium, ginkgo biloba, coenzyme Q10, bilberry, L-glutathione, soy isoflavones [genistein and daidzein], grapeseed extract, and green tea extract)

Take each of these twice daily, A.M. and P.M., with meals. (Dosage is suitable for individuals over twelve years of age.)

## 50. Do Eggs Have a Sunny Side?

You bet they do. They've been maligned, misunderstood, and mistreated, but they've made a nutritional comeback—and they've got a lot to offer. The American Heart Association, which formerly limited egg yolk consumption to no more than three per week, has changed its recommendation to no more than four egg yolks per week. It did this because new laboratory evidence showed that the dietary cholesterol in an average egg was 213 mg, not 274 mg as was previously thought. (This is not to say it upped its recommended guidelines on cholesterol consumption, which remains at no more than 300 mg of cholesterol per day.)

There is no controversy about the connection between cholesterol and heart disease. Innumerable studies have proven that your risk of heart attack increases when cholesterol levels in the blood become abnormally high. But whether eating eggs elevates serum cholesterol and triglycerides (blood fats) is another matter—one with enough cons and pros to fill a penitentiary.

## UNSCRAMBLING THE FACTS

- Lipoproteins are factors in our blood that transport cholesterol, and cholesterol behaves differently depending on the protein to which it is bound.
- Very low density lipoproteins (VLDL) have been found to bear a correlation to heart disease.
- High-density lipoproteins (HDL) are composed principally of lecithin, the detergent action of which breaks up cholesterol so that it is transported through the blood without clogging arteries. They have been found to help prevent heart disease.
- Eggs not only have the most perfect protein components of any food, but they also contain lecithin—and they *raise* HDL (the good cholesterol) levels!

| On the Down Side | On the Sunny Side |
|---|---|
| Some people suffer from a condition known as Type IV lipidemia, a hereditary inability to metabolize cholesterol. For them, eggs (despite their lecithin content) could still raise serum cholesterol levels. | Most people don't have this condition. |
| Many people, particularly children, are allergic to eggs. | Usually the egg whites (primarily albumen), not the yolks, cause the allergic reactions. |

Eggs are often fried in butter, bacon grease, and other saturated fats that can heighten the risk of heart disease and other ailments.

They can be fried without saturated fats in nonstick pans, or in pans lightly greased with unsaturated oil.

The FDA recently approved irradiating eggs to kill harmful bacteria such as salmonella, admitting that the process can lower nutritional content, particularly vitamin A.

Consumers can virtually eliminate the risk of salmonellosis by cooking eggs until the white sets and the yolk thickens. Salmonella is destroyed when kept at a temperature of 140°F for 3½ minutes or if it reaches 160°F. (See more egg safety suggestions below.)

They are easy to consume in excess, putting a strain on the kidneys to excrete the nitrogenous products of protein metabolism, which can also lead to a loss of calcium.

They're just as easy to consume in moderation, and better for you that way.

**NOTE** If you're allergic to eggs, you might also react adversely to products containing the additive lactalbumin phosphate. Check labels. It's frequently used in imitation dairy products, diet supplements, baked goods, frostings, breakfast cereals, fruit drinks, and sweet sauces, among others.

## EGG SAFETY SUGGESTIONS

- When purchasing eggs, look for grade A or AA eggs.
- Check eggs carefully and discard any that are cracked.
- Use eggs within thirty days of purchase.
- Store eggs in the refrigerator, at 40°F or below, in their original carton.

- Don't keep uncooked eggs unrefrigerated for more than two hours.
- Use pasteurized eggs in recipes that call for raw eggs, such as Caesar salad dressing or homemade ice cream.
- Don't eat raw cake or cookie batter.
- Be careful about eating scrambled eggs at brunch buffets. Restaurants sometimes combine eggs and a single bad egg can contaminate an entire batch.
- Always be sure that egg dishes served to infants, pregnant women, the elderly, or people with weak immune systems are cooked thoroughly. (See Chapter 11 for more on food safety.)

## 51. Cold Starters

Ready-to-eat cereals are plentiful, popular, and puffed up with nutrition claims. If they aren't boasting "less sugar," "good source of calcium," or "high fiber," it's "added nutrients" or "100 percent natural ingredients"—and they may still disguise nutritional shortcomings. Unfortunately, millions of Americans are swallowing these by the bowlful every morning.

**CONSUMER ALERT** Even some high-sugar, low-fiber cereals boast the American Heart Association's "Seal of Approval," but only because they are low in fat and have no cholesterol. Ridiculous! Nearly all cold cereals are low in fat, and *none* contain cholesterol!

### THE NAME GAME

Product names are often changed to make them appear more wholesome. For example, Post's Super Sugar Crisp is now Golden Crisp, though its 3½ teaspoons of sugar per serving are still the same. Kellogg's Sugar Frosted Flakes has slimmed down to Frosted Flakes, but the 2.8 teaspoons of sugar in its 1-ounce servings are still the same. And despite Sugar Smacks being transformed to Honey Smacks and now just Smacks, most of the cereal's sweetness still comes from sugar.

## THE HIDE-THE-SUGAR GAME

Simply because a cereal is low in sugar doesn't mean it is necessarily healthier for you. For example, whole-wheat Wheaties, called "the breakfast of champions," is low in sugar but contains 370 mg of sodium per ounce—not what I consider a winning way to start the day. In fact, many ready-to-eat cereals have been riding high on their low-sugar content while insidiously supplying more sodium per ounce than potato chips! A 1-ounce portion of Wise Potato Chips has approximately 190 mg of salt; a 1-ounce portion of Cheerios has 290 mg; Kix has 315 mg; Total and Kellogg's Corn Flakes have 280 mg. Children brought up on salty foods are more likely to become hooked on them in later life. And too much salt is just as much a health hazard as too much sugar (see section 110).

## THE PRESWEETENED MYTH GAME

Manufacturers claim that the reason they presweeten cereals—frequently to sugary levels of 3½ teaspoons per ounce—is to prevent consumers, particularly children, from adding too much sugar on their own. Now, really! How much more could they add? At this point, most presweetened cereals are little more than fortified candy. They might say they provide ten or more essential vitamins and minerals, but that doesn't mean you're getting them. Additionally, refined sugars (which presweetened cereals contain) deplete the body of B-complex vitamins, which are necessary for the proper assimilation of other vitamins and minerals.

Despite labels stating how many grams of sugar an ounce contains, few people realize what this figure converts to in teaspoons. An ounce of cereal is not a large portion, but it is considered a serving. And a single serving of a cereal such as Cap'n Crunch, for instance, with half a cup of milk, contains 18 g of sugar—*nearly 4 teaspoons!*

## THE FIBER–BRAN–BANDWAGON GAME

With substantial evidence that fiber can protect us from ailments ranging from constipation to cancer, manufacturers have jumped on the fiber–bran bandwagon with cereals galore. But all fiber is not the same (see section 116), and some of the most popular high-fiber cereals have enough sodium, sugar, and additives to counteract their potential benefits for many individuals. Hypertensives, diabetics, asthmatics, and anyone with gastrointestinal problems, for instance, should be aware that Kellogg's Fruitful Bran's 4 g of dietary fiber comes with 230 mg of sodium, 11 g of sugar, sulfur dioxide (see section 30), and sorbitol (see section 80), which may alter the absorption of some drugs, making them less effective or more toxic.

General Mills's Fiber One offers 12 g of dietary fiber, but is accompanied by 220 mg of sodium and contains aspartame (see section 81), which can adversely affect individuals with phenylketonuria (PKU), can elevate blood pressure, is contraindicated for anyone taking MAO inhibitors, and is not recommended for epileptics or pregnant women.

Post's Fruit & Fiber, which has 4 g of dietary fiber, is also not the best breakfast bet for asthmatics, allergic individuals, and hypertensives, since it contains sulfur dioxide, artificial flavors, and BHA.

Kellogg's Cracklin' Oat Bran, cashing in on the research that has shown the health benefits of soluble fiber (see section 116), contains more sugar than diabetics should have and four or more times as much fat as other cereals, with the exception of commercial granolas.

Despite their drawbacks, most dry high-fiber cereals have more nutrition benefits than other ready-to-eat cereals. But in order to reap these benefits, disregard advertising hype, read labels carefully, and select cereals that, for you, have the least amount of potentially harmful ingredients.

*Trade-Off Suggestions for Cold Cereals:* Preservative-free wheat flake and millet flake dry cereals. (Difficult to find in supermarkets, but worth a trip to your local natural food store.)

Unsweetened wheat germ, toasted or raw. (Toasted is tastier, but raw has more vitamins. To get the best of both, buy the wheat germ raw and toast it at home over a low flame in a dry pan. Refrigerate the unused portion in a tightly sealed jar.)

Homemade granola. (By making it without coconut, which contains a lot of saturated fat, and going easy on the oil and sweeteners, you can enjoy its nutritious benefits without compromising your health.) The following recipe makes about a pound and is as simple as it is delicious.

### GREAT GRANOLA

Heat 2 tbsp. honey, 2 tbsp. sunflower or sesame seed oil, and ⅛ tsp. vanilla. Pour this over a mixture of 1½ cups oats; ¼ cup wheat germ; ¾ cup chopped peanuts, almonds, and sesame, pumpkin, and sunflower seeds; and ¼ cup currants or raisins. Spread on shallow, flat pan and bake in a 325°F oven for 10 minutes. Stir to prevent sticking, then continue baking for another 10 minutes, or until toasty brown. (Serve with low-fat yogurt or applesauce.)

## 52. What's Hot and What's Not

Refinement might be socially commendable in people, but it is nutritionally reprehensible in cereals. In fact, the more refined grains are, the more reason for you to have less to do with them.

Whether a cereal has been dutifully enriched with synthetic replacements for lost nutrients or summarily degerminated (stripped of all but the kernel's starchy endosperm, then minimally reimbursed with synthetic substitutes), it is still refined—and capable of shortchanging you of important vitamins and minerals.

Many of these cereals are seductively appealing because they are quick-cooking, "instant" types; all the more reason to scrutinize labels and avoid those that contain disodium phosphate, an additive suspected of causing teeth and bone deterioration and kidney problems.

### NOT-SO-HOT CEREALS

Cream of wheat, cream of rice, farina, and hominy, which for years have been accepted as top-notch, high-nutrition hot breakfasts, are not, I'm sorry to say, the cream of the crop. All of them are degerminated—processed for creaminess by eliminating all grain germ and bran.

*Trade-Off Suggestion:* Whole-grain, stone-ground yellow cornmeal. It's as creamy as any of the cereals, but is not degerminated.

## THE HOT ONES

Oatmeal, with no sugar or salt, is an old-fashioned wholesome breakfast with a new plus going for it: oat bran, a soluble fiber that's been shown to help diabetics lower insulin requirements and aid in fighting heart disease by reducing serum cholesterol levels in low-fat diets.

Several oat bran cereals are now on the market. The best are those in which rolled oats, oat bran, or oat bran and another whole grain (wheat bran, wheat germ, and so on) are the only ingredients. The worst are highly processed (usually "instant"), and unhealthily endowed with natural and/or artificial sweeteners, sulfur dioxide, BHA, and a high sodium content. Such ingredients can negate the beneficial effects of oat bran, and post health risks for hypertensives and diabetics. (See section 116 for the differences between soluble and insoluble fiber.)

Cereals made with unrefined wheat, for example, Wheatena, are old standbys with a lot of contemporary nutritional merit (see section 130 for grains that do and don't make the grade), providing you don't subvert this by slathering them with sugar, butter, and salt. Admittedly, plain grain cereals without such flavorings are not appealing to modern taste buds, but they are healthier alternatives. I'm not going to tell you that these will be as tasty, because they won't. But they won't set you up for heart disease, diabetes, or arteriosclerosis, either—and, given a chance, they'll provide you not only with a way to enjoy more nutritious, and additive-free, foods more often, but, in many cases, to get extra vitamins and minerals as well.

| Instead of ... | Try Flavoring with ... |
|---|---|
| Refined sugar | Fruit juice, honey, raisins, fresh fruits (apricots, peaches, seedless grapes, strawberries), a dash of pure maple syrup or blackstrap molasses. (If you like blueberries, coat a handful with honey and then add them to your cereal for a fiber bonus and a |

|  |  |
|---|---|
|  | taste treat.) **CAUTION** If you are taking an anti-coagulant (blood thinner), don't use blackstrap molasses. It's high in vitamin K and can reverse the effect of your medication. |
| 1 tablespoon butter | 1 tablespoon low-trans or trans-free soft or liquid margarine; Benecol or Take Control margarine (see section 42); or peanut butter (no cholesterol and only 1.5 g saturated fat). |
| Salt | Cinnamon or nutmeg. |
| Whole milk | Low-fat or skim milk, or buttermilk; plain low-fat yogurt (add your own fresh fruit). |

## 53. Breads You Might Not Propose to Toast

Practically all breads you find in today's supermarkets have been processed and depleted of nutrients that are then replaced through *enrichment*—a euphemism if there ever was one. The standard of enrichment for white flour is replacing twenty-two natural nutrients with three B vitamins, vitamin D, calcium, and iron salts. That's not what I'd call enrichment, particularly since there is no guarantee that your body can utilize all, or any, of those added nutrients.

### WHITE BREAD

Regrettably still America's favorite, white bread is made from highly processed wheat flour that has been milled and bleached, and therefore depleted of numerous nutrients that enrichment cannot replace. Ironically, this has a redeeming feature. The processing causes the eradication of phytic acid, a chemical found in many whole grains that can prevent the body from using a number of minerals contained in flour. On the other hand, this is a dubious plus: Phytic acid has been found to help in the prevention of colon cancer. Weighing the pluses and minuses, the minuses have it.

- White bread contains mono- and diglycerides to maintain "soft-ness." Though present in small amounts, these glycerides can insidiously increase saturated fat intake because they are unknow-ingly being ingested regularly and frequently.
- Its formula is standardized by the Code of Federal Regulations and therefore the bread may contain more than a hundred food and chemical additives that need not be listed on the label!
- Even when made with unbleached flour, it is still lacking the two main constituents of the whole-wheat kernel: bran (the outer-most, vitamin B–rich fiber layer) and germ (the sprouting section that contains polyunsaturated fats, vitamin E, and other impor-tant nutrients).
- It can claim "no preservatives" and still contain dough condition-ers, such as potassium bromate (which has been known to cause central nervous system disorders and kidney problems) and sodium stearoyl lactylate, as well as chemical yeast nutrients such as calcium and ammonium sulfate (the former frequently used in wall plaster and the latter in fireproofing fabrics), among others.

**Minimize the Negatives**

- If you are going to buy white bread, at least make sure that it is enriched, and has the lowest sodium and fat, the most added nutrients, and no BHA.
- Buy thin-sliced, instead of regular, products.
- Choose breads made with unbleached flour over those made with white flour (often listed as "flour") or wheat flour, which is the same as white flour.
- Avoid commercial packaged breads with added calcium or sodium propionate (a bread made with quality ingredients under proper conditions doesn't need these added fresheners).

*Trade-Off Suggestions:* Hard-crusted, enriched Italian or French breads, which are soft and white inside, generally use unbleached flour and contain no sugar or animal fat. Pita breads, which are great for sandwiches, contain no sugar or shortening at all.

## DARK BREADS
### (Whole wheat, rye, oatmeal, pumpernickel, and so on)

Breads made from unrefined flour containing the entire bran, germ, and endosperm of grains are matchless sources of natural, life-sustaining nutrients. Unfortunately, most people never get to eat them. Modern milling processes and corporate profit quests have made their manufacture economically undesirable, and consumer gullibility has made it unnecessary.

Manufacturers have discovered that just about any brown bread packaged with words—particularly in old-fashioned lettering—such as "natural" (which may simply refer to specific ingredients) or "good source of fiber" (usually meaning little more than it provides 10 percent of the Daily Value of the reference food) can be passed off as nutritious. But until consumers wise up, the proverbial "staff of life" will continue to be just another flimsy stick. Just because a bread is dark does not necessarily mean that it's nutritious, or that it's the right bread for you.

- Many brown breads have little, if any, whole grains and are essentially white breads that have been colored with molasses.
- Dark breads are not inherently beneficial for all people. Breads made with whole wheat, rye, oats, and barley can worsen the health of individuals with celiac disease.
- Breads labeled "natural wheat" or "stone ground" may not be whole-wheat products. Unless "whole wheat" is listed as the *first* ingredient, the bread isn't.
- Wheat flour is *not* the same as whole-wheat flour. Actually, it is so far from it that it's virtually the same as bleached white flour—low in nutrients and full of chemicals.
- Some whole-grain breads use caramel color, which, despite its natural source, is a suspected carcinogen, and is under investigation for possible mutagenic properties.

### Minimize the Negatives

- Avoid breads made with hydrogenated shortening, dough conditioners, yeast nutrients, emulsifiers, or fresheners.
- Choose breads made with whole-wheat flour over others.
- Select loaves made with vegetable oil over those made with shortening. (Shortening is usually animal fat or partially saturated/hydrogenated vegetable fat and generally contains emulsifiers and other preservatives.)

## 54. Choosing Your Morning Bread Spreads

Whether it's a bagel, muffin, or just plain toast, what you spread on it daily for flavor can influence your well-being for life. Since so many breakfast spreads are high in saturated fats, cholesterol, salt, sugar, and additives—and are eaten frequently—discovering which ones are safest and healthiest for you is essential.

The butter versus margarine debate remains the one that has kept most people most confused ever since the *New England Journal of Medicine* reported that margarine posed cardiac risks of its own in the form of trans-fatty acids. But once you compare the unadulterated facts about both, I think you'll find it quite easy to make the right choice for your heart and your health.

### BUTTER

UNADULTERATED FACTS:

- The best butter is made from sweet cream and graded "U.S. Grade AA."
- One tablespoon of ordinary (not "sweet" or "unsalted") butter contains 100 calories, 11 g total fat, 7.1 g saturated fat, 3.3 g monounsaturated fat, 0.4 g polyunsaturated fat, 31 mg cholesterol, and 116 mg sodium.
- Salt helps preserve butter, but is often used to cover up off-flavors and staleness in inferior brands.

- Poor-quality butter (made from soured milk or cream with a lot of added salt to inhibit mold) often has an added alkaline salt to neutralize its salty taste.
- Virtually all commercial butters contain natural or artificial coloring, but need not state this on the label.
- Rancid butter can destroy fat-soluble vitamins in your body. (If it smells stale or looks odd, return it or throw it out.)

**COMMENTS AND CAUTIONS** If you use butter, use sweet, not salted, butter (you don't need extra sodium *and* saturated fat). I also advise using softened or whipped butter because it spreads more easily and you'll use less. Another way to minimize your intake of saturated fat is to blend butter with a quality soft or liquid margarine or with olive oil. You'll still have the butter flavor, but less cholesterol. (Gradually increasing the ratio of margarine to butter might help you make the switch.)

## MARGARINE

UNADULTERATED FACTS:

- Most margarines are made primarily from vegetable fat and oils that contain varying amounts of unsaturated fats. But when these are hydrogenated, or partially hydrogenated (to obtain the consistency of butter that is desired for marketing), they form unhealthy transfatty acids. *The harder the margarine, the more trans-fatty acids it contains.*
- Stick (solid) margarines contain trans-fatty acids which raise "bad" LDL cholesterol in the blood at least as much as the saturated fat in butter—and may also lower "good" HDL cholesterol.
- Functional food margarines, such as Benecol and Take Control, lower LDL cholesterol and raise levels of HDL cholesterol. (See section 42.)
- One tablespoon of regular margarine contains 100 calories (68 if whipped), 2.1 g saturated fat (1.4 g if whipped), 9 g unsaturated fat (6 g if whipped), 140 mg of salt (93 mg if whipped), and no cholesterol.

- With the exception of cottonseed oil (contained in virtually all "pure vegetable oils"), which has been exposed to more than a healthy share of chemical pesticides because cotton is not considered a food crop, the type of oil used is less important than how much it has been hydrogenated or hardened.
- Liquid vegetable oils low in saturated fats and high in polyunsaturates are best, provided they are listed as the products' *first* ingredient. Top in polyunsaturates are safflower oil (10 g per tablespoon), sunflower oil (8.9 g per tablespoon), soybean oil (8.1 g per tablespoon), and corn oil (7.8 g per tablespoon).
- If a label's first ingredient listing is any oil that has been partially hydrogenated or hardened, saturated fat predominates in the product.
- The softer the margarine, the less trans-fatty acids it has.

**COMMENTS AND CAUTIONS** All margarines contain additives, so read labels and avoid products containing any that might be potentially harmful to you (see sections 26 and 28). I'd suggest bypassing any containing EDTA, particularly if you are pregnant or on anticoagulant medication. If you are allergic to milk, Diet Mazola has no milk products and Mother's Sweet Unsalted Margarine has neither milk nor animal products. Avoid any margarines made with coconut or palm oil, which are more saturated than animal fat.

**SWEET SPREADS**
**(Jellies, jams, honey, fruit butters)**

UNADULTERATED FACTS:

- Most commercial jams and jellies are not made from fresh fruit. They contain canned, frozen, or strained extracts of frozen fruits.
- These products, with few exceptions, are more than half sugar, strictly refined, and sometimes combined with corn syrup. Honey is more expensive and rarely used, yet is the only sweetener that has to be listed on the label.

- Most fruit spreads contain benzoic acid or sodium benzoate (see section 26), artificial colors, flavors, and other additives. But because some of these are still not required to be listed, allergic individuals may be at risk.
- Jellies contain approximately 50 calories per tablespoon; jams and preserves approximately 55 calories; apple butter about 33 calories; honey has 64.
- Honey has more fructose than glucose and contains small quantities of minerals, as well as traces of B-complex vitamins and vitamins C, D, and E.
- Because honey is almost twice as sweet as cane or beet sugars, less of it is needed to achieve the same sweetness.
- Some manufacturers will add sugar syrup to their honey because it's cheaper and lightens the honey's color and flavor. (Be suspicious of inexpensive brands that are unusually thin when poured.)
- Some honeys may contain traces of penicillin and sulfites (creating danger for those who are sensitive), as well as cancer-causing substances that the bees extract from the flowers on which they feed.

**COMMENTS AND CAUTIONS** Sugar in any form poses serious health risks (see section 77) because we eat too much of it—more than 155 pounds per person a year! But if you are determined to have a sweet spread for your morning bread, I'd recommend honey over jam or jelly—although *not* for infants under the age of one year. (It may contain botulinum spores that their systems can't handle.) Because honey is sweeter, a little can provide a lot of flavor, without potentially harmful preservatives or vitamin-depleting refined sugars. Honey labeled "granulated," "creamed," or "spun" is best for spreading. (For more on honey, see section 80.)

Commercial jams and jellies have a lot of sugary negatives, but I don't advise replacing them with their artificially sweetened clones. These contain more potentially harmful additives, many of which don't have to be—and therefore, naturally aren't—listed on the label. You're better off using fruit butter as a spread, even more so if you make it yourself. There is nothing more to it than tossing diced organic apples, peels and all, into a pot, adding just enough water to prevent sticking, and simmering over a low flame for about an hour and a half, or until the pulp becomes dark and nicely thickened. An equally wholesome and quicker alternative is instant jam: Just mash some fresh berries with a little honey and you have your spread.

## CHEESY SPREADABLES
### (Pasteurized processed cheese spreads and cream cheese)

UNADULTERATED FACTS:

- With every ounce of pasteurized processed cheese spreads (ground and blended combinations of one or more natural cheeses), you get approximately 4 g of saturated fat, 16 mg of cholesterol, 81 calories, and 381 mg of sodium. But wait! That's not all. You also get an assortment of artificial colors and flavorings, stabilizers, optional acids, and a combination of more than one dozen different chemicals.
- One redeeming feature of these spreads (the only one) is that 2 tablespoons, approximately 1 ounce, contain more calcium (158 mg) than an entire cup of cottage cheese. But there are better calcium sources (see section 145), and certainly healthier ones.
- Cream cheese, made from fresh, dry, or concentrated milk and water, has a fat content in excess of 37 percent by weight. Whipped, it has approximately one-third less fat per tablespoon (but that's not by weight). In either form, that is a lot of fat.
- An ounce of cream cheese contains 100 calories, 6.2 g of saturated fat, 3.2 g of unsaturated fat, 31 mg of cholesterol, and 84 mg of sodium.
- Cream cheese is a poor source of protein and calcium (only 23 mg in an ounce).
- Many brands of cream cheese contain propylene glycol alginate (see section 26) and other additives that may pose potential health risks for you. Check labels carefully.

**COMMENTS AND CAUTIONS** If you feel that a breakfast bagel without cream cheese is unthinkable, try using Neufchâtel cheese. It tastes very much like cream cheese, but has a slightly lower fat content. Low-fat cottage cheese, too, is very spreadable and good for you. It can be sprinkled with chives for added zip. You might also want to try yogurt cheese, which is low in fat and wholesome on many levels. Be forewarned, though, that this cheese is tart. Then again, once you develop a taste for it, you're likely never to want cream cheese again.

As for using a pasteurized processed cheese spread, my advice is, don't. You are better off melting a thin slice of white cheddar, which will give you more protein, less sodium, and spare your body from having to cope with a barrage of chemicals the first thing in the morning.

## 55. Any Questions About Chapter 4?

*Do omega-3–fortified eggs really have omega-3 polunsaturated fatty acids? And how do they get in there?*

They really do have them, and they get in there the old-fashioned way—through the chickens' diet. Laying hens are fed a diet high in omega-3s, the fatty acids that have been shown to help lower cholesterol. Some producers use golden marine algae, a vegetarian source of docosahexaenoic acid (DHA) and eicosapentaenoic acid (EPA). Others supplement their hens' diets with flaxseeds or fish oils. The fortified eggs have between 50 mg and 150 mg of omega-3s per egg. This is a definite plus for eggs—and you—but not the way to get an adequate supply of omega-3s, which is 1,200 mg per day, into your diet. (You'd be consuming way more cholesterol than you want or need.) For the best ways to add omega-3s into your diet (without cholesterol), see section 112.

*If the amounts of trans-fatty acids aren't listed on labels, how do I know how much I'm getting?*

You don't. But you can look on the ingredient label for the words *hydrogenated* or *partially hydrogenated*. The lower down on the list these words appear, the fewer trans-fatty acids you're getting.

*Are there any breakfast cereals that kids would like that are low in sugar, non-GMO, and good for them?*

There are quite a few, although supermarket chains don't often carry them. Natural food stores are your best shopping bet. For instance, Mother's Natural Foods, a division of the Quaker Oats Company, has seven flavors of all-natural cold cereals that are sweetened with molasses or honey, including a peanut butter one formulated specifically for growing kids. New Organics is another company that has high-fiber, low-sodium organic cereals with a special line designed for children's tastes.

## FOOD FOR THOUGHT

- Most people think a bowl of cereal is one serving. It actually contains two or three times the amount of the serving size listed on the package label.
- If you're eating cottage cheese for breakfast to add extra calcium to your diet, you might not be doing so unless the brand is calcium enriched. Many low-fat and nonfat brands have had their liquid whey skimmed off, leaving only solid curds—and the whey contains most of the cheese's calcium.

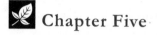 Chapter Five

# Coffee, Tea, or Milk?

### 56. That Not-So-Great Cup of Coffee

A lot of bad things have been said about coffee, and with good reason.

The "lift" you get from coffee that brings about an almost immediate sense of clearer thought and increased energy comes from the release of sugar stored in the liver. This is caused by caffeine, a central nervous system stimulant also present in tea, colas, chocolate, and some medications (see section 61). But it's an upper with a lot of downers:

> **Caffeine is one of the world's most psychoactive drugs.**

- As few as 3 or 4 cups of coffee daily can cause psychological and physical addiction.
- Depending on the amount consumed, or individual sensitivity, it can cause a condition known as caffeinism, with symptoms of appetite loss, irritability, insomnia, headaches, heart palpitations, stomach irritation, diarrhea, nausea, increased urination, anxiety attacks, flushing, chills, and, sometimes, a low fever.

- Caffeine's diuretic properties put extra stress on the kidneys and have a dehydrating effect on the body.
- Various studies have linked caffeine consumption to birth defects and the Center for Science in the Public Interest advises pregnant women to avoid it.
- The *American Journal of Obstetrics and Gynecology* reports that women who consume more than 150 mg of caffeine a day during pregnancy are more likely than those who consume less (or none at all) to miscarry between the third and seventh months of gestation.
- Effects of caffeine wear off less quickly on pregnant women and women on the Pill, taking about twice as long to clear out from their systems.
- Coffee increases the acidity in your gastrointestinal tract and can cause rectal itching.
- Drinking coffee to wake up in the morning can reset your body's circadian clock, interfere with your natural A.M. adrenaline, and cause a phase-delay similar to jet lag that can result in unexplainable drowsiness, depression, and insomnia, later on or the next day.
- Excessive intake of methylxanthines, a group of compounds to which caffeine belongs (and which includes theophyline, found in tea, and theobromine, found in chocolate), has been linked to fibrocystic breast disease and prostate problems.
- The British medical journal *Lancet* has reported a strong relationship between coffee consumption and cancer of the bladder and the lower urinary tract.
- Caffeine has been found to interfere with DNA replication.
- Studies at Stanford University have found that drinking 2 to 3 cups of strong coffee a day is associated with elevated cholesterol levels.
- People who drink 5 cups of coffee daily have a 50 percent greater chance of having heart attacks than those who do not drink coffee.
- Two cups of coffee can raise blood pressure about an hour after consumption, as well as decrease, then increase, heart rate.
- Caffeine can rob the body of B vitamins, vitamin C, zinc, potassium, and other minerals, as well as prevent the proper absorption

of iron; 5 (6-ounce) cups drunk within three hours can seriously deplete the body's supply of thiamine.

- The *American Journal of Clinical Nutrition* has reported that drinking 6 cups of unfiltered coffee a day causes a 10 percent elevation of blood levels of homocysteine (long associated with increased risk of heart attack and stroke), as well as a marked elevation in cholesterol levels and a 36 percent rise in triacylglycerols—both known precursors to artery-clogging atherosclerotic plaque.
- Caffeine concentrations in breast milk often rise above those in the mother's blood, frequently causing crankiness, insomnia, colic, and other symptoms of caffeinism in nursing infants.
- More than moderate caffeine consumption, over 300 mg daily, is inadvisable; excessive consumption, 1,000 mg (approximately 10 cups of coffee) daily, is risky; toxicity varies with individuals, but 10 g are estimated as the lethal dose.
- Abrupt abstention can cause mild to severe withdrawal symptoms.

Women who consume more than 400 mg of caffeine per day (about 4 cups of coffee) may be increasing their risk of urinary incontinence. According to a study from Brown University School of Medicine, caffeine appears to over-stimulate bladder muscles. The researchers suggest that all women limit caffeine intake and those with bladder problems avoid it completely.

## 57. The Dangers of Decaffeination

Just when you thought it was safe to drink coffee again, because each 5-ounce cup of brewed decaf contains only 3 mg of caffeine instead of regular's 115 mg, your health may still be jeopardized—and by something even more sinister: methylene chloride.

An acknowledged animal carcinogen (linked to liver and lung cancers), and a major pollutant (found in paint strippers), methylene chloride was the decaffeinating solvent of choice for seventy years. When it was discovered in the 1980s to have carcinogenic properties, most of the big U.S. coffee labels abandoned it. *But the Food and Drug Administration continues to permit the use of methylene chloride if the residues in the coffee are below 10 parts per million.* And, because it disturbs other flavorings so little, it is still widely used for specialty decafs. Though manufacturers claim that the solvent evaporates after the beans are steamed, heated, and blown dry, leaving only a tiny residue, 10 parts per million of a carcinogen ingested on a daily basis can mean big trouble brewing in you.

**COMMENTS AND CAUTIONS**  Flavored coffees often use propylene glycol (antifreeze) as a bonding agent. Although considered safe, it is an additive that you might not want to be consuming to excess. Also, some flavored coffees have shown the presence of other artificial compounds that are used for flavoring or as preservatives. A related concern is the use of dioxins and chlorine to bleach paper coffee filters. Natural unbleached filters are available and advisable.

## 58. Other Decaffeinators

There are safer, though more expensive, alternative methods for decaffeinating coffee. Products using them are well worth the price. Ethyl acetate, a natural derivative of coffee and fruits such as bananas and pineapples, is used to extract caffeine. The process takes more time, but the results are the same, only safer. Most teas use ethyl acetate for decaffeination.

Your wisest choice is to select brands that have been decaffeinated by the Swiss water process. No artificial chemicals are used in soaking the beans, which are later passed through activated charcoal or carbon filters to remove the caffeine. Products decaffeinated by the Swiss water process will say so; it's a sales plus of which manufacturers can be proud.

## 59. Withdrawal Warning

Weaning yourself from caffeine is not easy. In fact, studies have shown that heavy coffee drinkers can experience withdrawal symptoms twelve to sixteen hours after their last dose of caffeine, even if they've drunk decaf during that time period. The cutback in caffeine is substantial (see section 61 for comparisons) and the symptoms unpleasant.

But unpleasant as they are, if they're unrecognized for *what* they are, they can be confused with symptoms of other ailments, often resulting in misdiagnoses and unnecessary treatments. This does not mean that you should assume they are due to caffeine withdrawal and therefore ignore them. But if they coincide with your cutting back on caffeine, or making any dietary changes, your doctor should be informed.

## COMMON CAFFEINE WITHDRAWAL SYMPTOMS OF WHICH MOST PEOPLE ARE NOT AWARE

- Headaches (eliminating a habitual after-dinner cup can cause morning headache the next day; tension headaches are often caused by recurrent caffeine withdrawal; holiday and weekend headaches occur frequently in office workers used to regular coffee breaks during the workweek)
- Irritability (sudden anger, intolerance of ordinary occurrences, frustration)
- Depression (moodiness, bouts of crying, general apathy, disinterest in work and hobbies, social withdrawal)
- Runny nose
- Nausea, queasiness, and vomiting (intermittent, frequently confused with stomach viruses)
- Fatigue (yawning, drowsiness)
- Dizziness

Easing up on caffeine should be done gradually. (A good way to start is by brewing equal parts regular and decaf, then increasing the proportion of decaf to regular.) Though some people can do it in a day or two with no repercussions, most require at least two weeks.

## 60. Coffee Trade-Offs

There are two main species of coffee beans—*Coffea Arabica* and *Coffea Robusta*. Arabicas have approximately half the caffeine content of Robustas, which are less expensive and used when more caffeine is wanted. (Most decaffeinated coffees, for example, are made from Robustas because they provide a larger amount of caffeine for resale to manufacturers of soft drinks and drugs.)

| Instead of ... | Switch to ... |
| --- | --- |
| Regular coffee | "Light coffee" (a blend of wheat or chicory and coffee, with a generally lower caffeine content) |
| Drip coffee | Percolated (has approximately 30 mg less caffeine) |
| Percolated coffee | Instant (has approximately 15 mg less caffeine) |
| Instant coffee | Brewed decaffeinated (has approximately 62 mg less caffeine) |
| Brewed decaffeinated coffee | Instant decaffeinated (has approximately 63 mg less caffeine) |
| Instant decaffeinated coffee | Grain beverages, such as Postum or Pero (which are sort of imitation coffees made from bran, wheat, and molasses), or Cafix (made from barley, rye, chicory, and beets), have no caffeine. |

**CAUTION** Though these grain products are low in calories and caffeine free, excessive consumption may have an unwanted laxative effect or cause flatulence.

If you crave a caffeine lift but want to avoid caffeine consequences, try ginseng (see section 132) or fruit juice, the natural sugar content of which can give you an energy boost with a vitamin bonus.

## 61. Caffeine Comparisons to Keep in Mind

The following table has been designed to give you perspective regarding caffeine consumption and help you keep yours at a safe 300 mg daily. You're likely to find that you are getting more caffeine jolts than you think.

| Coffee | Per 5-Ounce Serving |
|---|---|
| Dripolated | 110–150 mg |
| Percolated | 64–124 mg |
| Instant | 40–108 mg |
| Light coffee-grain blend | 12–35 mg |
| Decaffeinated | 2–5 mg |
| Instant decaffeinated | 2 mg |

| Tea | Per 5-Ounce Serving |
|---|---|
| Black 5-minute brew | 20–50 mg |
| Green 5-minute brew | 35 mg |
| Black 3-minute brew | 20–46 mg |
| Black 1-minute brew | 9–33 mg |
| Instant | 12–28 mg |
| Iced | 22–36 mg |
| Decaffeinated (see section 57) | 10–41 mg |

| Chocolate | |
|---|---|
| Cocoa (5-ounce cup) | 4–6 mg |
| Milk chocolate (1 ounce) | 5–6 mg |
| Dark chocolate, semisweet (1 ounce) | 20–35 mg |

| Soft Drinks | Per 12-Ounce Serving |
|---|---|
| Jolt Cola | 74 mg |
| Mountain Dew | 54 mg |
| Mello Yello | 52 mg |

| Soft Drinks | Per 12-Ounce Serving |
|---|---|
| Diet Mr. Pibb | 52 mg |
| Tab | 46 mg |
| Coca-Cola | 46 mg |
| Diet Coke | 46 mg |
| Shasta Cola | 46 mg |
| Dr. Pepper | 44 mg |
| Pepsi-Cola | 41 mg |
| Diet Pepsi | 38 mg |
| RC Cola | 36 mg |
| Mr. Pibb | 33 mg |
| 7 UP | 0 mg |
| Root beer | 0 mg |
| Ginger ale | 0 mg |
| Decaffeinated colas | trace |
| Tonic water | 0 mg |
| Club soda, seltzer | 0 mg |

| Drugs | Per Tablet |
|---|---|
| Vivarin | 200 mg |
| Bio Slim T Capsules | 140 mg |
| Aqua-Ban | 100 mg |
| Cafergot | 100 mg |
| NoDoz | 100 mg |
| Excedrin | 65 mg |
| (Excedrin P.M. has no caffeine but does have an antihistamine) | |
| Fiorinal | 40 mg |
| Vanquish | 33 mg |
| Anacin | 32 mg |
| Darvon Compound | 32 mg |
| Empirin | 32 mg |

| Drugs | Per Tablet |
|---|---|
| Midol | 32 mg |
| Soma Compound | 32 mg |
| Triaminicin | 30 mg |
| Aspirin | 0 mg |

## 62. The Tea Alternatives

The amount of caffeine in tea varies according to the type of leaves and the strength of the brew. The longer tea steeps, the more caffeine it will have. The average cup has about half the caffeine of coffee, and loose teas contain much less than tea bags.

Be forewarned that decaffeinated teas still contain some caffeine. Lipton decaffeinated tea has only 10 mg, but Salada has 41 mg. For caffeine-sensitive individuals, 3 or more cups daily could cause adverse reactions.

All herbal teas can contain caffeine, so it's important to read the labels. Celestial Seasonings Morning Thunder, for instance, the flavor of which is derived from mate (a South American plant with leaves rich in caffeine) and other tea leaves, contains 35 mg of caffeine. Flavored black teas (orange, cinnamon, blackberry, apple, and so forth) contain about the same amount, which is still less than unflavored black teas. Some decaffeinated flavored teas, such as those made by Bromley and Benchley, have about 24 mg per tea bag.

Caffeine-free herbal teas make fine, caffeine-free alternatives to coffee, but they do have other hazards of which you should be aware. (See section 119.)

**COMMENTS AND CAUTIONS** Whether you drink coffee or tea, decaf or regular, don't drink it hot! Drinking hot beverages—above 157°F—may significantly raise your risk of esophageal cancer. (The *International Journal of Cancer* reported that people who drank more than 2 cups of hot beverages daily over the course of several years *quadrupled* their risk of this cancer.) Keep in mind that you can burn your mouth on liquids as low as 140°F, and restaurants often serve coffee at 170 to 190°F, so let it cool down to 125°F, or until it doesn't burn your tongue before you take a sip.

## 63. What Could Be Wrong with Milk?

A lot if . . .

- You're an adult concerned about your fat consumption, because whole milk has 65 percent saturated fatty acids and only 4 percent polyunsaturates.
- You or a member of your family has a lactose intolerance (a deficiency of the enzyme lactase, necessary for milk digestion), which can cause such gastrointestinal problems as bloating, cramps, bad breath, and diarrhea; or a milk allergy, essentially a *casein* allergy (hypersensitivity to the protein in milk), which can cause reactions such as breathing difficulty, serious stomach pain, eczema, asthma, ear infections, excessive fatigue, diarrhea, or constipation, among others.
- You are concerned about arteriosclerosis (an acknowledged precursor to heart attacks), because the fatty particles in homogenized whole milk can pass through the stomach wall into the bloodstream, making arteries susceptible to cholesterol buildup.
- You consider that the FDA does not ban the use of BGH (bovine growth hormone), which increases milk production but can leave potentially harmful residues in milk.
- You have stomach acidity problems or ulcers. Studies show that milk stimulates gastric acid secretions and aggravates rather than soothes ulcerative or preulcerative conditions.
- You have hypertension or cardiovascular disease and want to keep your sodium intake in check. Milk and all milk products, with the exception of low-sodium milk and cheeses, supply a lot of sodium.
- Your children drink it in place of other, iron-rich foods. Overconsumption of cow's milk, a poor source of iron, can cause

microscopic losses of blood from the gastrointestinal tract and lead to iron-deficiency anemia.

- The milk is raw (unpasteurized), because it may contain dangerous microorganisms that could cause serious illness, and be potentially lethal for infants, young children, the elderly, and anyone with a compromised immune system.
- It has an off-flavor that could be caused by cow feed sprayed with harmful pesticides.
- You rely on it as your sole source of calcium. Adults and growing children need 800 to 1,200 mg of calcium daily. Three 8-ounce glasses of whole milk will give you only 776 mg of calcium—not enough and certainly not worth the 360 mg of sodium, 33 mg of cholesterol, 15 g of saturated fat, and 577 calories you'll get with it. Exchanging whole milk for skim or low-fat milk, or buttermilk, will cut back calories and fat, but still won't provide enough calcium. (See section 145 for additional sources.)

**COMMENTS AND CAUTIONS** The FDA allows drug-contaminated milk to be sold as long as the residues are at a "safe" level. These so-called "safe" levels have been shown to cause increases in drug-resistant strains of bacteria that cause virulent diseases.

## 64. Milk Trade-Offs

### IF YOU HAVE A LACTOSE INTOLERANCE

- Lactaid milk, which is lactose free. Available as whole milk or fat free.
- Lactaid Ultra—caplets that are taken before eating dairy that enable the body to digest and break down lactose.
- Lactaid Extra—chewable caplets that are taken before eating dairy and enable the body to digest and break down lactose.
- Acidophilus milk—uses safe bacterial cultures, such as those in cheeses, yogurt, and sour cream, to predigest the lactose.
- Buttermilk—made with skim or low-fat pasteurized milk to which a bacterial culture that predigests lactose is added.

- Sweet acidophilus milk—bacterial cultures are added, but don't break down the lactose until the milk enters your digestive tract. This milk cannot be warmed, used for cooking, or added to hot liquids.

## IF YOU HAVE A MILK ALLERGY

- Soy milks.
- Dairy products marked "parve"; these are milk free.
- Water or Rice Dream (rice milk) can be substituted in cooking recipes. For baking, you can also substitute fruit juice (but reduce the amount of sugar called for in the recipe).

**COMMENTS AND CAUTIONS** Any food item may be processed on equipment that has previously processed a dairy product, and the equipment may carry residual dairy material, so there is a risk of cross-contamination. Also, many brands of canned tuna fish contain "hydrolized caseinate." Always read ingredient labels.

Remember that *nondairy* does not mean milk free, and that medicines and vitamin supplements may also contain milk products, so be sure to ask your pharmacist.

Avoid products that contain curds, whey, casein, sodium caseinate, lactalbumin (most all ingredients beginning with *lact*), recaldent (found in some chewing gums), and chicken broth (many brands contain milk solids). Many "natural ingredients" may also contain dairy products; check with the manufacturer.

## TO MINIMIZE CHOLESTEROL AND SATURATED FAT

- Skim milk (4 mg cholesterol, 0.28 g saturated fat per cup).
- Buttermilk (9 mg cholesterol, 1.3 g saturated fat per cup).
- Mix 2 percent milk with skim milk (you will get a lot more taste and only a little more cholesterol and fat).
- Use soy milk. It's lactose free and cholesterol free.

- Use sour cream instead of heavy cream.
- Use soy milk instead of cream when cooking—you get the rich texture of real cream, but without the real fat.
- Use sour half-and-half, or low-fat yogurt, instead of sour cream.

## TO MINIMIZE SODIUM

- Low-sodium milk (95 percent of the sodium has been removed).

## FOR THE CREAM IN YOUR COFFEE

- Mix equal parts whole milk and skim milk; better yet, use equal parts low-fat (or 2 percent) and skim milk.

## 65. Never Trust a Nondairy Creamer

Keep your glasses with you when you shop so that you can read the small print on nondairy creamer labels. You'll be in for quite a few surprises.

- Though these "creamers" don't contain lactose, almost all contain sodium caseinate, a derivative of milk protein that can cause reactions in people with milk allergies. Moreover, the processing used to produce sodium caseinate results in the formation of lysino-alanine (LAL), which is under investigation as a factor in causing kidney damage, and, if spray-dried, may also result in the formation of nitrites (see section 49).
- Nondairy does not mean either "low calorie" or "unsaturated fat." Despite their lack of butterfat, the primary fat source in these "creamers" is almost always a highly saturated vegetable oil (such as coconut oil, which is more saturated than most animal fats) that supplies as many calories as and usually even more saturated fat than whole milk.
- Many nondairy creamers also contain carrageenan, an additive that can interfere with the body's immunological warning system and should be avoided.

- Nondairy creamers have no nutritional value worth mentioning, and can contain up to 68 percent sugar.
- Liquid creamers usually have more calories per serving, but generally have substantially lower levels of saturated fat.
- A few nondairy creamers use soy protein instead of sodium caseinate, but beware of those that merely claim to contain a nonspecific vegetable protein.

## 66. Any Questions About Chapter 5?

*I drink low-fat milk all the time and have gotten to the point where it tastes the same as whole milk to me—except in my coffee. Does the coffee cause the milk to change?*

No, it's the other way around. A milk's fat content produces the change in coffee's color (the reflecting of light from homogenized fat globules causes the coffee to look lighter). It is essentially an optical effect. If someone else adds the milk to your coffee, and you don't look at it before you drink it, you'll find that you no longer taste the difference.

*I have a milk allergy and was told to avoid foods that are labeled "high protein" or "protein enriched." Why is that?*

The added protein in these foods is usually a version of another ingredient, such as wheat, and the version used is often milk protein.

*My six-year-old daughter is allergic to milk. She eats no dairy products at all, and I'm concerned about her getting enough calcium in her diet for her growing bones. Are there good nondairy sources of calcium?*

There are lots more than most people imagine. Just ½ cup of cooked spinach, for instance, contains 130 mg calcium. And 3 ounces of canned salmon (with bones) supplies 180 mg of calcium. Other good sources are almonds, tofu, beans, sardines, kale, collard greens, soybeans, and molasses. There are also calcium supplements that come in chewable form, but be sure to avoid any that contain calcium lactate (which is a milk sugar derivative); calcium gluconate is okay because it comes from a veg-etable source.

## FOOD FOR THOUGHT

- Milk from BGH-injected cows may contain residues of more than eighty different drugs, many of them antibiotics, used to treat sick animals. As disease organisms are exposed to these antibiotics, they become increasingly resistant to drug treatment. Well over ten thousand people die in the United States each year due to antibiotic-resistant strains of bacteria.
- One cup of Ben & Jerry's No Fat Coffee Fudge Frozen Yogurt has 85 mg of caffeine!

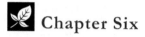 Chapter Six

# The Lunch Crunch

### 67. Dying for Lunch?

Two heart attacks occur every minute in the United States. The top nutritional culprits, according to a study conducted by the Department of Health and Human Services, are fat, cholesterol, sodium, and sugar. If you think you have cut your risk of cancer and heart disease just because you no longer eat butter or use cream, have virtually eliminated fried foods from your diet, trim the fat from your meat, drink diet sodas, and haven't had bacon or sausage with your eggs for years, you are fooling yourself and foiling your health. *It's not so much a matter of what you do or don't eat, but rather how often you do or don't eat it that matters!*

### 68. Packing Lunch Boxes with Trouble

White bread and rolls (see section 53) provide large portions of unwanted nutrients because we eat them so often. But they are the frame for sandwiches and account for 22.3 percent of our combined fat, sodium, and sugar intake before we even put anything on them.

Since bread alone does not a sandwich make, add any of the following and you'll have a pretty good idea of what else you're getting:

| Filling | Fat | Sodium |
|---|---|---|
| Bologna | 11 g | 737 mg |
| Ham | 17 g | 476 mg |
| Turkey (white meat) | 2.2 g | 42 mg |
| Swiss cheese | 15.6 g | 148 mg |
| American cheddar cheese | 18.8 g | 352 mg |
| Peanut butter | 36 g | 298 mg |
| Tuna fish (water packed) | less than 1 g | 216 mg |

Add a tablespoon of mayo, butter, or margarine and you'll have another 11 g of fat. (That's also 140 mg of sodium if you use butter or margarine; mayo has only 14 mg.) A tablespoon of mustard and ketchup, on the other hand, will spare you the fat, but the mustard will give you 195 mg of sodium and the ketchup an equally substantial 156 mg, as well as more sugar than an equivalent portion of ice cream!

Also, with the exception of bratwurst, virtually all luncheon meats, frankfurters, knockwurst, and other processed meats, as well as smoked fish, contain nitrates and nitrites (see section 49).

## 69. Sandwich Cautions

Stocking up on fillings, or preparing sandwiches beforehand so you can get the kids off to school or yourself off to work in time, is a fine idea, providing you keep a few things in mind.

### SANDWICH SAFETY

- Even if refrigerated, don't keep uncured luncheon meats for more than four to seven days. (If they get that shiny, slimy look, toss them out.)
- When making sandwiches with uncured meats, don't let them stand unrefrigerated for more than 5 to 10 minutes. (Rewrap and refrigerate quickly to prevent bacterial growth.)

- If you are making chicken, egg, or tuna fish salad, refrigerate immediately after adding the mayonnaise. (The mayo itself doesn't spoil, but when combined with tuna, chicken, hard-boiled eggs, or meat, it can become a bacterial spawning ground.) You can keep the sandwich cold until lunchtime by packing it with a box of frozen juice or a "Blue Ice" pack.
- If making a sliced egg or egg salad sandwich, be sure not to let the cooked unshelled eggs cool in water. (Cooling eggs in water causes them to lose their natural protective layer and sets up a breeding ground for bacteria that produce a nerve-damaging toxin. If they are then stored in airtight containers, even more toxins are produced.) The best way to cool boiled eggs is to let them stand in the open air and then refrigerate them.
- Make sandwiches on frozen bread. This will keep the filling cool and the sandwich will taste freshly made when lunchtime arrives.
- Sandwiches can be made ahead of time and frozen (wrapped in foil) until needed. But lettuce and other greens should not be frozen; they can be added when the sandwich is taken out of the freezer.

## 70. The Scoop on School Lunches

School lunches, though nutritionally balanced in theory, are in fact so nutritionally poor (with very few exceptions) that they are virtually hazardous to a growing child's health. Although these meals are required to provide at least one-third of a child's recommended daily nutrient allowance (by including milk, a protein-rich food, fruit, vegetables, a grain food, and butter or margarine), they rarely do. Most of the meals are low in fiber, high in refined carbohydrates and sugars, and surfeited with processed, vitamin-depleted foods. And adding insult to nutritional injury, the food tastes awful, too, as evidenced by what gets tossed in the lunchroom garbage.

Additionally, many schools have vending machines for gum, soft drinks, and other junk foods, which compound the problem by teaching children poor nutritional habits right in their halls of learning.

The convenience of having a child eat a school lunch is not worth the nutritional cost. A high-sugar intake at lunch can cause a drop in blood sugar during the afternoon, which can in turn leave a child fatigued, inattentive, and unable to retain what is being taught. Refined sugar has also been linked to delinquency. (See section 151.)

## 71. Simple Sandwiches for Superior Performance

It is easier than you think to prepare nutritious lunches for your child and yourself without having to resort to expensive, nonnutritive processed luncheon meats.

### SEVEN SUPER SANDWICH LUNCHES YOU CAN PACK IN PLAIN BROWN BAGS

1. Cottage cheese and (unsweetened) pineapple sandwich on nut bread/carrot sticks/sunflower seeds/low-fat milk.
2. Tuna salad with lettuce in pita bread/cherry tomatoes/pear or peach/low-fat milk. (Yogurt can be used instead of mayo for making tuna salad and is just as good, and it has much less fat.)
3. Ricotta (or cottage) cheese and raisin sandwich on banana bread/green pepper slices/tangerine/low-fat milk.
4. Peanut butter and sliced apple sandwich/carrot sticks/orange slices/low-fat milk.
5. Chicken salad with chopped celery in pita bread/apple/low-fat milk.
6. Baked beans (mashed with a little onion and homemade chili sauce) in pita bread/cucumber strips/melon slices or cubes/low-fat milk.
7. Chopped egg (mixed with a little mayo or yogurt, grated onion, and carrot) on oat bread/peanuts/grapes/low-fat milk.

## 72. Fast-Food Foolishness

Lunch is the meal most people eat away from home, and eating at fast-food restaurants has become a national pastime, as well as a shortcut to widespread health problems.

I'm not condemning fast foods as nutritional wipeouts. They have a few (and I mean a *few*) redeeming features, primarily protein (see section 107). And an occasional burger and fries (and I do mean *occasional*) is unlikely to cause any serious repercus-

> **If you think the four major food groups are McDonald's, Burger King, Pizza Hut, and Wendy's, you are in trouble.**

sions for most people. But if you think that the four major food groups are McDonald's, Burger King, Pizza Hut, and Wendy's, you are in trouble.

The biggest problem with fast foods is their abundance of saturated fat and sodium. Since heart disease is the nation's number one killer, the fact that many fast-food chains still fry their food in shortening that is largely beef tallow (it's hard to get fat more saturated than that), and have excessive amounts of salt in everything, is undeniably scary.

Consumers are generally unaware of how much fat and sodium they are getting because they don't expect it in things such as shakes (Burger King's vanilla has 9 g of fat and 329 mg of sodium) or apple pie (a serving at McDonald's has 19 g of fat and 414 mg of sodium). But it's there. And if you have a Whopper and fries with your Burger King shake you are getting a total of 51 g of fat and 1,243 mg of sodium—and that's without dipping your fries in ketchup (at 156 mg of sodium per tablespoon) or sprinkling them with salt. No matter what your age or gender, that's more fat and sodium than your body can handle for lunch—or any single meal—on a regular basis.

## 73. Fast-Food Calorie Countdown

| Burgers | Calories |
| --- | --- |
| Burger King Whopper | 663 |
| McDonald's Big Mac | 587 |
| Hardee's Big Deluxe | 557 |
| Wendy's Single (w/cheese) | 547 |
| Jack-in-the-Box Jumbo Jack (w/out cheese) | 544 |

## Burgers                                    Calories

| Burgers | Calories |
|---|---|
| Arby's Cheeseburger | 492 |
| Roy Rogers ¼ lb. (w/cheese) | 416 |

## Chicken                                    Calories

| Chicken | Calories |
|---|---|
| KFC Crispy Dinner (3 pieces of chicken) | 950 |
| KFC Original Recipe Dinner | 830 |
| Jack-in-the-Box Chicken Supreme | 572 |
| Roy Rogers Fillet Sandwich | 526 |
| KFC Original Sandwich w/sauce | 450 |
| Wendy's Fillet Sandwich | 441 |
| KFC Original Sandwich w/o sauce | 360 |
| McDonald's McNuggets (3¾ oz.) | 286 |

## Fish                                       Calories

| Fish | Calories |
|---|---|
| Long John Silver's Fish Sandwich | 560 |
| Hardee's Big Fish | 515 |
| Burger King Whaler | 502 |
| Arthur Treacher's Fish Sandwich | 440 |
| McDonald's Fillet-o-Fish | 373 |
| Long John Silver's Fish (2 pieces) | 318 |

## Pizza and Tacos                            Calories

| Pizza and Tacos | Calories |
|---|---|
| Jack-in-the-Box Super Taco | 375 |
| Taco Bell Taco Light | 372 |
| Pizza Hut Thick 'N Chewy Pepperoni Pizza (¼ of 10-in. pie) | 280 |
| Pizza Hut Thin 'N Crispy Cheese Pizza (¼ of 10-in. pie) | 225 |
| Taco Bell Taco | 194 |
| Jack-in-the-Box Taco | 174 |

## Other Entrées                                          Calories

| | |
|---|---|
| Arby's Roast Beef Sandwich | 416 |
| Roy Rogers Ham/Swiss | 416 |
| McDonald's Egg McMuffin | 352 |
| Dairy Queen Cheese Dog | 330 |
| Hardee's Chili Dog | 329 |
| Wendy's Chili (small) | 310 |
| Roy Rogers Roast Beef Sandwich | 298 |

## Fries (small)                                          Calories

| | |
|---|---|
| Wendy's | 317 |
| Long John Silver's | 282 |
| McDonald's | 268 |
| Roy Rogers | 230 |
| Kentucky Fried Chicken | 221 |
| Jack-in-the-Box | 217 |
| Hardee's | 202 |
| Arby's | 195 |
| Burger King | 158 |

## Chocolate Shakes                                       Calories

| | |
|---|---|
| Roy Rogers | 518 |
| McDonald's | 377 |
| Burger King | 367 |
| Wendy's | 367 |
| Arby's | 365 |
| Jack-in-the-Box | 324 |
| Hardee's | 273 |

## 74. Some Fast-Food Fat Trade-Offs

If you're going to eat fast foods, you might want to give some heartfelt
thought to choosing the lesser of their fatty evils.

| Instead of . . . | Consider Perhaps . . . |
|---|---|
| KFC Extra Crispy Dinner (3 pieces of chicken), which contains 54 g fat | Pizza Hut Thin 'N Crispy Cheese Pizza (¼ of 10-in. pie), which contains 7.5 g fat |
| Burger King Whaler with 46 g fat | Two pieces of Long John Silver's Fish with 19 g fat |
| McDonald's Big Mac with 31 g fat | Taco Bell Taco with only 8 g fat |
| Cheeseburgers | Regular burgers |
| Fries | Coleslaw |
| Fried clams, shrimp, or oysters | Large pieces of fish (which have more food in proportion to batter); or even better, broiled fish |
| Fried chicken | Broiled chicken; or removing the batter-fried skin |
| Shakes | Fruit juice |

Learn to balance fast-food indulgences with a subsequent meal containing fresh fruit, green and yellow vegetables, whole grains, beans, and foods that are rich in vitamins A and C, the B complex, and iron. (For a list of the best sources, see section 145.)

## 75. Not-So-Hot Dogs

Hot dogs might have made Nathan's famous, but they won't do much for you.

### A HOT DOG BY ANY NAME IS STILL NOT SO HOT

- Its main ingredient is the scraps and trimmings of muscle meat, usually beef and pork (unless otherwise stated), but not necessarily in equal proportions or in that order.

- It consists primarily of water and (mostly saturated) fat: approximately 56 percent water and 26 percent fat.
- It contains preservatives and flavorings, such as salt, sweeteners, ascorbic acid, sodium erythorbate or ascorbate, and nitrite.
- Sodium content ranges from 300 mg (Best's Kosher Beef Lower Fat hot dog) to 645 mg (Hygrade's Beef hot dog).
- According to the Cancer Prevention Coalition, children eating a dozen hot dogs a month have nine times the risk of getting leukemia as the average child.
- Pregnant women eating one or more hot dogs a week double the risk of brain tumors for their babies.
- Frankfurters can contain *Listeria monocytogenes,* a potentially fatal bacterium particularly harmful to pregnant women, newborns, people with weakened immune systems, and the elderly.

**MY ADVICE** The next time you decide you want to eat a hot dog, change your mind. But if you just can't say no to hot dogs, *make sure that they're cooked until they're steaming hot!*

## 76. Any Questions About Chapter 6?

*What's the worst thing about fast foods?*

Aside from people eating them too often, they contain too much protein, salt, fat, and calories and not enough complex carbohydrates and fiber. One typical fast-food meal (cheeseburger, fries, and shake) can supply 90 percent of your daily protein, and often a day's worth of fat, salt, and calories as well. This leaves little leeway for healthful eating, and plenty of room for extra pounds of trouble.

*My husband is a truck driver, and he eats a lot of fast foods, even though he sometimes develops a rash after eating them. Do you know what causes this? And are there any vitamins that can help?*

A lot of fast-food ingredients can trigger allergic reactions in sensitive individuals. Along with such additives as FD&C Yellow No. 5 (often in hotcakes and milk shakes), corn sugar (frequently in French fries), and milk solids (used in fish fillets), MSG is probably the most frequent culprit. It has been known to cause rashes, itches, and insomnia in individuals with no previous allergies or food sensitivities. And most fast-food restaurants use MSG, particularly in soups, but also in burgers and other foods.

Another possibility could be sulfites, which though now banned from being sprayed on fresh vegetables, are still used in frozen ones, soups, potato salad, gravies, beer, and foods commonly served at diners and fast-food restaurants. (See section 32.)

I'd suggest your husband take a high-potency multiple vitamin and mineral, twice daily (with meals), that contains vitamin C (500 mg), vitamin E (200 to 400 mg), and vitamin B complex (50 to 100 mg). I would also take 1 to 3 MSM tablets (1,000 mg) two to three times daily. And considering his eating habits, one multiple digestive enzyme with meals is also recommended.

## FOOD FOR THOUGHT

- A typical fast-food hamburger contains meat from dozens or even hundreds of cattle.
- Chicken McNuggets contain beef extracts. And McDonald's French fries, although cooked in vegetable oil, derive their flavor from beef products that are sprayed on them before they are deep-fried.
- A single animal infected with *E. coli* can contaminate 32,000 pounds of ground beef.
- French fries are the most frequently listed food item on kids' menus offered at the nation's top 500 chain restaurants. Out of 1,937 items, salad appears only eleven times.
- Recent research has linked soft drinks with childhood obesity— and an estimated two hundred school districts nationwide have contracts with soft-drink companies that give them exclusive rights to sell their products in schools.

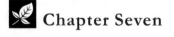 Chapter Seven

# Scary Snacks

### 77. The Unsweet Side of Sugar

We are eating 11 more pounds of sugar, or its equivalent, than we did ten years ago, when we were eating 118.1 pounds of it annually! What's worse is that most of us don't even know it.

All carbohydrate sweeteners qualify as sugar, even though they may be called by other names (see section 13). And sugar is often found in products we wouldn't think contained it, such as salt, peanut butter, canned vegetables, bouillon cubes, medicines, toothpaste, vitamins, and more.

**WHAT SUGAR CAN DO TO YOU**

- Cause tooth decay, loss of essential nutrients, and mood swings, and contribute to obesity.
- Aggravate asthma, mental illness, and nervous disorders.
- Increase the possibility of heart disease, diabetes, hypertension, gallstones, back problems, arthritis, hypoglycemia, and other ailments.
- Potentiate salt to raise blood pressure and imbalance the body's calcium/phosphorus ratio.

## 78. A Table of Sugar Contents

With sugar, it is definitely a matter of hide-and-sweet, since manufacturers know that consumers do not desire its presence. Yet sugar, which provides none of the forty-four nutrients needed to sustain life, accounts for more than 24 percent of the calories the average American consumes daily, whether he or she knows it or not.

| FOOD | SERVING SIZE | APPROXIMATE TEASPOONS OF SUGAR PER SERVING |
|---|---|---|
| **Drinks** | | |
| Birds Eye Awake | 4 oz. | 3 |
| Canada Dry Tonic Water | 12 oz. | 8¼ |
| Chocolate milk | 8 oz. | 6 |
| Cola beverages | 12 oz. | 10 |
| Eggnog | 8 oz. | 8 |
| Ginger ale | 6 oz. | 5 |
| Grapefruit juice (unsweetened) | 4 oz. | 2½ |
| Hi-C Orange Drink | 6 oz. | 5 |
| Kool-Aid | 8 oz. | 6 |
| Malted milk shake | 10 oz. | 5 |
| Orangeade | 8 oz. | 5 |
| Orange juice | 4 oz. | 2½ |
| Root beer | 10 oz. | 4½ |
| 7 UP | 6 oz. | 3¾ |
| Tang | 4 oz. | 4 |
| **Candies** | | |
| Chewing gum | 1 stick | ½ |
| Chocolate bar | 1½ oz. | 2½ |
| Chocolate mints | 1 | 2 |

| FOOD | SERVING SIZE | APPROXIMATE TEASPOONS OF SUGAR PER SERVING |
|------|--------------|---------------------------------------------|
| **Candies** | | |
| Granola clusters | 1 oz. | 3½ |
| Gumdrop | 1 | 2 |
| Hard candies | 4 oz. | 10 |
| Lifesavers | 1 | ⅓ |
| Marshmallows | 1 regular | 1½ |
| Milky Way | 1 oz. | 4 |
| Peanut brittle | 1 oz. | 3½ |
| **Cakes, Cookies, and Pies** | | |
| Angel food | 1 4-oz. piece | 7 |
| Apple pie | 1 slice | 12 |
| Brownie | 1¾ oz. | 3 |
| Cheesecake | 1 4-oz. piece | 2 |
| Cherry pie | 1 slice | 14 |
| Chocolate cake (plain) | 1 4-oz. piece | 6 |
| Chocolate cake (iced) | 1 4-oz. piece | 10 |
| Chocolate cookie | 1 | 1½ |
| Chocolate éclair | 1 | 7 |
| Cream puff (iced) | 1 regular | 5 |
| Cupcake (iced) | 1 | 6 |
| Doughnut (plain) | 1 | 3 |
| Doughnut (glazed) | 1 | 6 |
| Fig Newtons | 1 | 5 |
| Gingersnaps | 1 | 3 |
| Macaroons | 1 | 6 |
| Oatmeal cookies | 1 | 2 |
| Pumpkin pie | 1 slice | 10 |
| Sponge cake | 1 4-oz. piece | 1½ |
| Sugar cookies | 1 | 1½ |

| FOOD | SERVING SIZE | APPROXIMATE TEASPOONS OF SUGAR PER SERVING |
|---|---|---|
| **Fruit and Dairy Desserts** | | |
| Applesauce (unsweetened) | ½ cup | 5 |
| Canned fruit cocktail | ½ cup | 5 |
| Canned peaches in syrup | 2 halves (1 tbsp. syrup) | 3½ |
| Chocolate pudding | ½ cup | 4 |
| Ice cream cone | 1 | 3½ |
| Ice cream soda | 1 | 5 |
| Ice cream sundae | 1 | 7 |
| Sherbet | ½ cup | 9 |
| Tapioca pudding | ½ cup | 3 |

## 79. Why Quick Pickups Let You Down

Simple sugars, which most candies are, require little metabolizing and enter your bloodstream quickly, giving you that much-touted lift. But the catch is that your pancreas, the organ in charge of releasing insulin to process carbohydrates (starches and sugars) to keep blood sugar at a steady and healthy level, is caught off guard by the sudden surge of sugar, and, thinking it has more work to do than it has, releases too much insulin. The result is an in-body processing error that lets you down the hard way: a drop in blood sugar, usually within an hour, that leaves you feeling less energetic, less alert, and more hungry and irritable than you were before you ate the sugar.

## 80. All Sugars Aren't the Same

There is no doubt that a sugar by any name is still a sugar (even when it is called a carbohydrate), but that doesn't mean they are all the same, or hazard free.

## SUGAR REVIEWS THAT AIN'T SO SWEET

**Sucrose**   This is refined white table sugar, granulated or powdered, made from either sugarcane or sugar beets. Though a disaccharide, meaning a double sugar (composed of glucose and fructose, in this case), it is totally lacking in protein, vitamins, and minerals. The B vitamins needed for its assimilation must be obtained from other foods or supplements; when ample B vitamins are not supplied, they are taken from the body and can cause deficiencies.

**Glucose**   The body's blood sugar, glucose is also found in most fruits. It's a monosaccharide, the simplest form of sugar in which a carbohydrate is assimilated. It is rapidly absorbed and can upset blood sugar balance in the same way as sucrose, though it is only half as sweet. It is one of the basic sugars in sweeteners.

**Dextrose**   Dextrose is a monosaccharide that is chemically identical to glucose (which is frequently referred to as dextrose) and made from cornstarch.

**Fructose**   Also known as levulose, this is a natural sugar found in fruit. It is preferred to sucrose because the body absorbs it more slowly. But many fruits are mainly sucrose, so fructose should *not* be considered safe for diabetics or hypoglycemics. Additionally, the fructose used in foods is usually the result of enzymes added to corn syrup, which produces sucrose that is then further processed into high-fructose corn syrup. Even when derived solely from a natural source, fructose is a highly refined product and, like sugar, is devoid of nutrients.

Because fructose is sweeter than sucrose, and less is needed to obtain the same sweetness, it is often used in "lite" products to reduce calorie content by the necessary one-third. This has its advantages for weight watchers, but is not without drawbacks: Large amounts of fructose can cause diarrhea and gastrointestinal pain. It has also been found to cause a marked elevation in cholesterol levels.

**Maltose**  This is a disaccharide made from the malting of whole grains. (Sounds nutritious, but it isn't.) Though not nearly as sweet as either sucrose or fructose, maltose is much less likely to cause cavities.

**Lactose**  This is milk sugar, a combination of glucose and galactose, and the least sweet of all. Despite its derivation from milk, it is as nonnutritive as all other refined sugars, and can cause adverse reactions in individuals with a milk allergy or lactose intolerance. (See section 63.)

**Brown Sugar**  This is just plain old white refined sugar with molasses coloring.

**Raw Sugar (Also known as "natural," blond, and turbinado sugar)** Raw sugars are all simply white sugar, packaged at 96 percent sucrose; table sugar is bleached and purified to 99 percent. You might pay more for them, but you are still getting nothing but empty calories—and no nutritional benefits to offset the cost.

**Blackstrap Molasses**  The liquid that remains after beet or cane sugar has been thoroughly processed and the sucrose has been removed is blackstrap molasses. Though still 65 percent sucrose, blackstrap molasses contains minor but useful amounts of iron, calcium, potassium, and B vitamins, particularly vitamin $B_6$. Lighter molasses is less endowed with nutrients.

**CAUTION**  If you are under levodopa treatment for Parkinson's disease, blackstrap molasses is not recommended.

**Sorghum Molasses**  This is a lighter molasses, made from sweet sorghum (a cereal grass in the millet family). The juice is extracted from sorghum stalks through crushing and is then boiled down into syrup. Unless the syrup is heated properly it may quickly ferment in the jar. Most manufacturers add enzymes to make it more stable. In any event, iron is its only significant nutrient, and the product is still about 65 percent sucrose.

**Barbados Molasses**  This is another light molasses, processed the same way as sorghum, only sugarcane is used instead of sorghum. Its taste is much like blackstrap molasses, only more palatable, but it has virtually none of blackstrap molasses's nutrients. (**Note:** No molasses or any other sweetener made from sorghum or sugarcane is organic, since neither is considered a food crop and the plants are frequently sprayed.)

**Honey**  This nectar of the gods is still sugar and has the highest calorie content of all natural sweeteners, approximately 65 calories per tablespoon. (Refined sugar has only 48 calories per tablespoon.) Honey does have small amounts of potassium, calcium, and phosphorus, which is more than you can say about refined sugar; and truly natural honey that is only heated to low temperatures (just enough to remove beeswax and other impurities) contains natural enzymes and pollen, a rich source of protein.

But consumers are being stung by honey rip-offs. Now that honey has become popular with the health conscious, manufacturers heat it to high temperatures to give it a crystal-clear purity that sells well, but destroys nutrients. Some suppliers feed their bees sugar water, or worse, add sugar syrup to their honey for a better flavor.

Unfortunately, everything about honey isn't sweet. Not only can it rot teeth faster than sucrose, various honeys have been found to contain carcinogens that bees have extracted from flowers sprayed with cancer-causing pesticides. And some kinds of honey (as well as corn syrup) can be fatal to infants, whose digestive tracts aren't mature enough to prevent the growth of the botulinum spores that are occasionally present in these sweeteners.

**Maple Syrup**  If you want a naturally really sweet sweetener, pure maple syrup is one of the best, but it is expensive. Nonetheless, like molasses, maple syrup is still 65 percent sucrose, so no matter how much or little you pour on pancakes or French toast, approximately half is the equivalent of white sugar. Unfortunately, not all 100 percent pure maple syrup is 100 percent safe. Some producers don't make their maple syrup the old-fashioned way—by gathering the sap in lead-free buckets, boiling it down over hardwood fires, and bottling it. Instead, formaldehyde pellets are used to keep the tap holes from healing and increase sap flow. (Ingestion of formaldehyde, which is used in embalming fluids, can cause severe abdominal pain, internal bleeding, nausea, inability to urinate, coma, and death.) They also gather the sap in lead-soldered buckets. (The adverse effects of lead on infants and young children can occur at very low levels, causing symptoms ranging from mild anemia to severe brain damage and death.) Additionally, they boil sap over oil fires, filter it, and add chemical antifoaming or polishing agents. Since all syrup tends to foam during processing, cream or animal fat may be used to reduce this, although some producers now use natural vegetable oil. (If you want to be sure the product contains *no* animal fat, check the ingredients or look for the word *parve* on the label.)

**Malt Syrups**   Nutritionally superior but not as sweet as maple syrup, malt syrups are made from cereal grains (barley, rice, and wheat) and contain mainly maltose and glucose sugars. Keep in mind, though, that just because these syrups aren't as sweet as others doesn't mean they have a lower sugar content. Watch out for malt syrups that add sweetness with commercial corn syrup, which is industrially refined glucose.

The least sweet, but most wholesome, is 100 percent barley malt syrup. Rice syrup or rice honey, which is a mixture of barley and rice, comes in two types: one 20 percent barley and 80 percent rice, the other mostly rice with grain enzymes. Unfortunately, neither barley nor rice syrups are made from totally organic grains.

**Xylitol**   Though found naturally in berries, fruits, and mushrooms, xylitol is produced commercially from "wood sugar," or xylose. Generally extracted from birch cellulose (a birchwood by-product of the plywood industry), it is considered a carbohydrate alcohol. It has the same caloric value as sugar, but is metabolized differently and therefore used in products for diabetics and hypoglycemics. Also, because bacteria in saliva don't grow on and ferment xylitol—as they do other sugars—to produce cavity-causing acids, it is used in many sugar-free chewing gums, hard candies, cough syrups, and oral hygiene products such as toothpastes, lozenges, and mouthwashes.

Until 1986, the only known adverse effect of large doses of xylitol had been diarrhea. But some research showed that large doses, in long-term feeding studies, caused tumors and organ injury to animals; additionally, humans receiving xylitol intravenously as an energy source experienced liver, kidney, and brain disturbances. Therefore, it had to be reevaluated. After review, it was FDA approved as an additive for use in foods for special dietary needs. In 1996, the Joint Expert Committee on Food Additives (JECFA) confirmed that adverse findings in earlier animal studies were "not relevant to the toxicological evaluation . . . in humans." The JECFA has allocated an Acceptable Daily Intake (ADI) of "not specified" for xylitol. (ADI, expressed in terms of body weight, is the amount of a food additive that can be ingested daily over a lifetime without risk.) An ADI of "not specified" is the safest category in which JECFA can place a food additive. The Scientific Committee for Food of the European Union (EU) also deemed it "acceptable" for dietary use. It's unacceptable as far as I'm concerned, and excessive intakes can still cause diarrhea.

**Sorbitol**   Half as sweet as sucrose, sorbitol (known as a sweet alcohol) occurs naturally in fruits, berries, algae, and seaweeds. But these are not the sources manufacturers use. It is made industrially from hydrogen and commercial glucose (corn sugar). Because of its slow absorption into the bloodstream, it is also used in sugar-free gums (see section 82), candies, and other products okayed for use by diabetics and hypoglycemics. It does, though, have a laxative effect, and large doses (or frequent ingestion) generally cause diarrhea.

**Mannitol**   Much like sorbitol, this sweet alcohol occurs naturally in beets, celery, and olives. It can be derived from the manna plant or seaweed, but is made industrially from hydrogen and glucose (corn sugar). Only half as sweet as sucrose, it is often used in powdered products, such as the dusting on chewing gum and breakfast cereals. It has a laxative effect at lower levels than sorbitol, and may produce diarrhea quite easily in infants and young children.

**Stevia**   This is an herb that is two hundred times sweeter than sugar. A natural sweetener, stevia has no calories, is suitable for diabetics, and is available as a powder or liquid at health food stores.

## 81. Real Facts About Artificial Sweeteners

Once upon a time, artificial sweeteners were used primarily by diabetics, who cannot adequately metabolize carbohydrates and for whom sugar can be lethal. Today, more than seventy million Americans, less than half of them diabetics, consume products containing sugar substitutes—none of which have been shown to be (at best) more than a partial aid to weight control and all of which pose health risks.

### SACCHARIN

One of the earliest commercially used artificial sweeteners in the United States, saccharin is a noncaloric petroleum derivative estimated to be three hundred to five hundred times sweeter than sugar, though it has a bitter aftertaste (usually masked by the addition of the amino acid glycine). Absorbed, but not modified by the body, it is excreted unchanged in the urine. It's used in diet soft drinks, toothpaste, and medicines, and is available as the sugar substitute Sweet 'N Low.

Studies done in the 1970s linked saccharin ingestion to bladder cancer in laboratory animals. The FDA proposed a ban on its use in 1977, but protests from consumers and the American Medical Association, the American Society of Internal Medicine, the National Academy of Sciences, the American Diabetes Association, and others called for a moratorium on the ban. While the moratorium was in effect, warning labels informing consumers of the laboratory tests and the possibility of cancer were required on all products containing saccharin. On December 22, 2000, saccharin was removed from the National Toxicology Program's

(NTP) report on carcinogens and warning labels are no longer required on foods containing it. For diabetics, who must restrict carbohydrate intake, saccharin might be worth taking. For the general public, it's not a sweetener that I would recommend.

## CYCLAMATE

Noncaloric and thirty times sweeter than sugar, cyclamate is less expensive than either saccharin or aspartame. Previously banned in the United States and Britain, because of studies showing that when mixed with saccharin it increased the risk of bladder cancer, the JECFA has now approved it as safe for humans at specified levels, although some countries still restrict its use.

## ASPARTAME

Technically not an "artificial" sweetener because it is composed of two amino acids (phenylalanine and aspartic acid) that are natural components of many common proteins, aspartame contains as many calories per gram as sugar (4 g) but is about two hundred times sweeter, so much smaller amounts are needed. It is considered safe by the FDA and AMA except for persons suffering from phenylketonuria (PKU), an inherited inability to metabolize phenylalanine that can lead to severe retardation. (Phenylalanine can interfere with the body's chemical neurotransmitters that conduct nerve impulses within the brain. Children who drink large quantities of diet sodas containing aspartame are particularly vulnerable to its dangerous side effects.) Marketed as NutraSweet, it has replaced saccharin in almost all diet soft drinks, with the exception of Dr. Pepper. It is used in an enormous variety of dietetic and low-calorie products, as well as medicines, and is available as the sugar substitute Equal.

Aspartame contains methyl or wood alcohol, which can affect fetal brain development. I would advise pregnant woman who are watching their weight to avoid using diet products containing aspartame or any artificial sweetener.

**CAUTION** If left on a shelf at a warm temperature over a period of time, the chemical in the artificial sweetener aspartame breaks down into formaldehyde, a known carcinogen. If you must drink diet colas sweetened with aspartame, don't drink them frequently, use them by their sell-by date—and keep them cool.

## 82. What Four Out of Five Dentists Don't Tell You About Sugarless Gum

Four out of five dentists might recommend sugarless gum for their patients who chew gum, probably because they don't know what the fifth dentist does: that sugarless gum, or candy, can increase your chances of tooth decay if it contains sorbitol or mannitol—which most of them do.

Although neither sorbitol nor mannitol itself promotes cavities, both of them nourish and increase the type of bacteria in your mouth—namely, *Streptococcus mutans*—that do. According to Dr. Paul Keyes, founder of the International Dental Health Foundation, *Streptococcus mutans* have the mechanism to stick to teeth but will remain harmless until you eat something containing sugar or sucrose, with which they then quickly combine to cause decay. Because the sorbitol and mannitol have swelled the ranks of these bacteria, there are more of them available to use passing sugars to attack your teeth.

If you can't brush after every sweet, you can fight back by rinsing your mouth with water immediately (within fifteen minutes) after eating or drinking anything that contains sucrose.

### OTHER TOOTH-SAVING TIPS

- Eating aged cheese—cheddar or Swiss—can reduce the ability of plaque to form cavity-causing acids.
- Have your sweets *with* instead of *between* meals. (Sweets eaten with meals have little tendency to cause decay.)

- Be sure you are getting enough iron in your diet (see section 145), since sugars cause more damage to teeth if the body is deficient in iron.
- Increase your intake of fibrous foods (vegetables, whole-grain breads and pasta, cereals) that promote a stronger saliva flow and, essentially, "rinse" your teeth more frequently.
- Avoid excessive consumption of acidy fruit juices, which can wear away tooth enamel.
- Choose puddings or ice cream (which can be easily rinsed from the mouth) over caramels or fudge-type candies that stick to the teeth and are difficult to remove.
- If you are going to have a sweet, treat yourself and your teeth to a *small* piece of chocolate. Despite its multiple nutritive negatives, chocolate has been found to have decay-inhibiting properties.
- And try kissing more often. It stimulates the salivary glands, the saliva helps rinse food particles away, and, though it's not as effective as brushing or flossing, it's certainly more fun.

## 83. The Sweet Treat That Ought to Be Behind Bars

It is not difficult to become a chocoholic, but it is not healthy, either. In fact, chocolate's few benefits are far outweighed (in more ways than one) by its nutritional hazards.

### THE GOOD CHIPS ABOUT CHOCOLATE

- It can help inhibit tooth decay. (Chocolate liquor, in chocolate candy, when mixed with sucrose, has been found to neutralize the effect of sucrose on the mouth's decay-causing bacteria, reducing their ability to produce cavity-causing acids.)
- It contains phenylethylamine, a natural mood-elevating substance that the brain produces when you are in love—and craves when you fall out of it. It may also boost the brain's production of serotonin, a natural antidepressant.

**NOW THE BAD . . .**

- Chocolate, made from the cacao bean, contains significant amounts of caffeine (see section 56), which is an addictive drug.
- It is capable of depleting inositol, which aids in the redistribution of body fat, promotes healthy hair, and can help prevent eczema and keep cholesterol levels low.
- It can prevent the proper absorption of calcium, needed for the body to metabolize iron, and therefore diminish energy, reflexes, bone strength, and disease resistance; aggravate insomnia; and promote irregular heartbeats.
- It can deplete the body of vitamin $B_1$ (thiamine) and other B vitamins needed for fighting stress and aiding carbohydrate digestion.
- Its caffeine content can put heavy stress on the endocrine system, particularly a child's, and deplete necessary stores of potassium and zinc.
- It can delay the healing of canker sores.
- It is contraindicated for—and should definitely be avoided by—anyone who has herpes.
- It can worsen allergy symptoms and decrease the effectiveness of antihistamine medicines.
- It can decrease the effectiveness of tranquilizers, sedatives, and relaxants.
- It can cause serious hypertension in anyone taking MAO inhibitors or antidepressants.
- It has a large number of empty calories in small portions, making it easy to fill an empty stomach with too much fat and too few nutrients.

## 84. The Candy–*Candida* Connection

Yeast infections *(Candida albicans)* occur when the *Candida,* or yeast organism, gets out of control in the body, producing a toxin that not only affects the nervous system (causing headaches, fatigue, depression, hyperactivity, and memory loss, among other symptoms), but also the reproductive organs, leading to abdominal pain, persistent vaginitis, bladder problems, loss of sexual interest, and more.

Antibiotics, nutritional deficiencies, diabetes mellitus, birth control pills, cortisone, anxiety or physical stress, improper hygiene, chronic constipation or diarrhea, and food or chemical allergies are all possible causes of yeast infections, which are curable—provided you don't undermine the cure with the wrong foods.

*Candida* needs certain foods to survive. This often causes patients suffering from yeast infections to experience overwhelming cravings for sweets, on which *Candida* thrives. Giving in to these cravings will keep *Candida* multiplying, along with producing uncomfortable side effects.

## FOODS TO AVOID

To eliminate yeast infections, avoid sugar, refined carbohydrates, all yeast-containing foods, and any foods that may have mold; particularly, candy, ice cream, chocolate, chewing gum, colas, dried fruits, cheese, raised breads, sour cream, buttermilk, beer, wine, cider, soy sauce, vinegar, frozen or canned juices, mushrooms, tofu, and melons.

## FOODS TO INCREASE

Some foods are natural combatants for yeast infections, and increasing them in your diet can help. Among them are garlic, onions, broccoli, cabbage, plain yogurt, turnips, and other vegetables.

## A HELPFUL SUPPLEMENT REGIMEN

- An all-natural, high-potency multiple vitamin and amino acid–chelated mineral complex (containing no preservatives or artificial colors), A.M. and P.M.
- A broad-spectrum antioxidant formula (containing alpha- and beta-carotene, lutein, lycopene, vitamin C, vitamin E, selenium,

gingko biloba, coenzyme Q10, bilberry, L-glutathione, soy iso-
flavones, grapeseed extract, and green tea extract), A.M. and P.M.
- Vitamin C, 1,000 mg (time release), A.M. and P.M.
- Vitamin E (dry form), 200 to 400 IU daily
- Propolis, 500 mg, three times daily

## 85. Little Snacks Can Have Big Dangers

There is no harm in having a snack or two now and then, unless you think
of *now* as today and *then* as tomorrow, and wind up having one or more
daily. Even the calories in little snacks add up quickly. Just one pack of
Lifesavers, eaten every day, can put 10 pounds on you in a year. And
there's a lot more to being overweight than not fitting into your old jeans.

### OBESITY

- Shortens life expectancy
- Increases the risk of diabetes, heart attacks, strokes, gout, respiratory diseases, arthritis, and more
- Has been found to be a factor in female infertility, menstrual
  disorders, toxemia, and various forms of cancer
- Can delay wound healing, lower resistance to infection, and
  generally undermine the body's immune system

## 86. There's Nothing Bright About Artificial Colors

Artificial coal tar–based (azo) dyes have been used extensively as colorings
in snack foods and confections for years, though not without objection.
Seventeen have finally been banned, delisted, and deemed hazardous by the
FDA, but a tenacious seven—FD&C Red No. 3, Blue No. 1, Blue No. 2,
Green No. 3, Yellow No. 5, Yellow No. 6, and Red No. 40—remain.

Four of these have been shown to cause cancer and brain tumors in
laboratory animals. Three are under investigation for safety because of
assorted findings of toxicity in research studies. All are still being used to
color our foods.

**SOME DYE-HARD SNACKS TO THINK TWICE ABOUT**

Fruit drops, fruit Jell-O, Kool-Aid, caramels, Lifesavers, fruit drinks, filled chocolates (not pure chocolates), most flavored ice cream, maraschino cherries, fruit-flavored Popsicles, flavored soda, pie fillings, "penny" candies, many fruit yogurts, caramel custard, puddings (vanilla, butterscotch, and chocolate), crackers, cheese puffs, virtually all artificially colored candies

If you are allergic to aspirin, are asthmatic, or suffer from eczema, be forewarned that foods containing azo dyes are more likely to affect you adversely. (See section 28.)

# 87. Assorted Unappetizing Snack Additives

**CARRAGEENAN**

This is a suspected carcinogen, possibly a factor in ulcerative colitis; most harmful when taken in a beverage. Frequently used in chocolate products, pressure-dispensed whipped cream, cheese foods, ice cream, frozen custard, sherbets, ices, jellies, and jams.

**DEXTRANS**

This is a suspected carcinogen; most often used in soft-centered candies.

**XYLITOL**

See section 80.

**HYDROGENATED/PARTIALLY HYDROGENATED COCONUT, PALM KERNEL, OR RAPESEED OIL**

These are highly saturated fats. They are used in candy bars, malted milk balls, fruit chews, cookies, crackers, baked confections, whipped toppings, and fruit punches.

## MODIFIED FOOD STARCH

This may be a factor in calcium deposits in kidneys and growth retardation. The type of starch used is rarely identified; used in crackers, cookies, muffins, candies, marshmallows, and fruit punches.

## CONFECTIONER'S GLAZE

This is refined shellac made for food use by bleaching regular shellac that's used on furniture. No long-term feeding studies on safety have been done. It's used as a coating for many candies and baked confections.

See section 26 for acacia gum, alginates, BHA, BHT, propyl gallate, and others.

## 88. Smarter Snack Trade-Offs

| Instead of ... | How About ... |
|---|---|
| Potato chips or pretzels, both of which are veritable mines of salt (pretzels have 495 mg per ounce) and can deplete you of B vitamins, while offering you no nutritional benefits and taxing your liver unfairly. | Popcorn. It is filling instead of fattening (only 41 calories per ounce), a great source of fiber, and if you sprinkle it with some debittered yeast (not brewer's yeast) instead of salt, you'll have a terrific snack with nutrients galore. |
| Salted peanuts, which are roasted in oil and high in fat, sodium, and calories. | Shelled or unshelled dry unsalted roasted peanuts. You eliminate the sodium and still benefit from protein and B vitamins. Raw peanuts should be cooked quickly at a high temperature in the oven or a nonstick pan |

| Instead of . . . | How About . . . |
|---|---|
| | before eating. This destroys a substance in them that can otherwise interfere with the body's ability to metabolize essential nutrients. |
| Commercial tortilla chips, such as Doritos, which are made with the most saturated of hydrogenated oils (coconut, palm, and cottonseed) and contain 7 g of fat per ounce, along with a roster of unwanted additives, including MSG, FD&C Yellow No. 5, and gum arabic, and can turn snack time to allergy attack time. | Homemade tortilla wedges. Stack five 8-inch flour tortillas and cut into eight wedges to make forty chips. Spread these in a single layer on two baking sheets, bake for ten to fifteen minutes at 375°F, or until crispy. Instead of 7 g of fat, you'll get only 1—and no unnecessary additive side effects. |
| Chocolate, which has numerous strikes against it. (See section 83.) | Carob, the powdered seed of the carob tree. It has a flavor similar to chocolate but contains no theobromine or caffeine—and is much lower in fat. |
| Ice cream, which is often filled with hidden and potentially harmful additives (see section 26) and has more fat than you need. | Low-fat yogurt sweetened with fresh fruit or a bit of honey; frozen sherbet; frozen juices made into additive-free Popsicles. |

## Instead of ...

Nonnutritive, chewy caramel
candies, which are usually filled
with additives and are being
investigated by the FDA for
nitrogen-containing impurities
that might be present in caramel
manufactured by an ammonia
process.

A hot dog or hamburger,
both of which have numerous
nutritional drawbacks.
(See sections 72 and 75.)

Fast-food shakes, with their high
fat and additive content.

Chewing gum, which aside from
containing empty calories,
unwanted additives, and artificial
colors and flavorings, stimulates
the saliva that prepares the
digestive tract for food it doesn't
receive, as well as creating
increased hunger and
gastrointestinal problems.

## How About ...

Dried fruits. (See section 142.)
They are as sweet as candy
and good sources of vitamin A
(ten dried apricot halves supply
more than 3,000 IU) and calcium
(raisins have 18 mg per ounce).

A taco or a slice of pizza. These
can offer more in the way of
vitamins, minerals, and complex
carbohydrates and less in the
way of fat.

Homemade shakes. (Fruit plus
¾ cup powdered milk, ½ cup
orange juice, and 1½ cups water
with a few ice cubes makes a
shake that can be kept cold in a
thermos, or frozen and eaten like
a Popsicle.)

Raw carrots and celery sticks.
These satisfy your urge to chew
and provide wholesome, health-
promoting vitamins and minerals,
particularly vitamin A, vitamin C,
calcium, phosphorus, and
potassium, as well as many
essential amino acids.

| Instead of ... | How About ... |
|---|---|
| Sweets of any kind. | Sunflower seeds. These can actually suppress your urge for sweets (as well as cigarettes, by the way). They release glucose from the liver, which then rushes to the brain like adrenaline and produces a similar "lift" effect. The calories are still there (406 in ½ cup), but they offer plenty of protein (17.5 g), no cholesterol, 5.2 mg of iron, and a good 87 mg of calcium. |

## 89. Any Questions About Chapter 7?

*I've recently started a diet, and to curb my appetite, I have taken to chewing gum. But I've noticed that after chewing, the blood vessels in my face seem to become redder. Have you any idea why?*

I would suspect that the gum contains BHT (see section 26), which frequently causes allergic reactions. Try not chewing gum for a day and keep away from all products containing BHT. If your facial redness doesn't disappear, consult your doctor immediately.

*I've read that manufacturers are not required to list all the additives in ice cream because it's a standardized food. Are any of the additives in it harmful, and is there any way for me to find out which ice creams have the least amount?*

All additives are *potentially* harmful. As a rule, the cheaper brands use more synthetic ingredients. Any containing piperonal, often used as a substitute for vanilla (as well as a chemical to kill lice); ethyl vanillin, which has caused liver, kidney, heart, lung, and spleen damage in laboratory animals; butyraldehyde, which gives a nutlike flavor to ice cream (and is also an ingredient in rubber cement); and isoamyl acetate, a banana-pear flavor used in many ice creams (and several shoe polishes) are ones I would strongly suggest you avoid.

An ice cream with few additives should melt slowly to form a custardlike cream, not watery liquid. To test, put the edge of a spoon into softened ice cream. When you pull it out, the ice cream should stick to the spoon. If the spoon comes out clean, the ice cream contains more additives than you want.

**I've heard of a natural sweetener called amasake. What is it, and is it safe?**

Amasake is similar to malt syrups, but it is made from cooked rice, barley, or other grain, and inoculated with *Aspergillus oryzae* mold (koji), which turns grain starch into sugar. It is not recommended for diabetics. Since *Aspergillus* is a fungus source suspected of producing carcinogens during metabolism, I'd say it is a risky sweetener at best and recommend avoiding it. Use stevia instead. It's available as a powder or liquid extract from the leaves of the stevia shrub. It's much sweeter than sugar (using too much can produce a bitter flavor), and it is suitable for diabetics. For the equivalent of 1 cup of sugar you need only ½ to 1 teaspoon stevia. You'll find it at health food stores.

**I'm trying to lose weight and cut back on sugar, but I get throbbing headaches from aspartame. Is there another sugar substitute I could try?**

There is Splenda, which is made of sucralose, which comes from sugar, and is therefore somewhat better from a health standpoint than other artificial sweeteners. Although it says it has no calories, there are 2 calories per teaspoon. (This is allowed under current labeling laws.) It's fine for sweetening beverages, but according to *Consumer Reports* it is not recommended for baking.

**I was told I'd be better off eating real potato chips than fat-free ones. I thought the less fat the better, so how can this be?**

It can be because most fat-free potato chips and snacks contain the fake fat Olestra. This synthetic fat (also known as Olean or sucrose polyester) was designed so that it couldn't be broken down by the body's enzymes and would, therefore, not be absorbed by the body. Great in theory but not in fact, because Olestra has some very unwanted side effects. Aside from the widely publicized "brown stain" effect (from many people experiencing loose stools and fecal urgency), it depletes the body of fat-soluble vitamins A, D, E, and K, as well as carotenoids. And although Olestra is now fortified with these vitamins, it's only to the government's determination of the minimum amount to prevent deficiency—certainly not to maximize health. (Early studies found that just six chips a day could reduce a person's beta-carotene level by 50 percent!) True, Olestra will reduce the total grams of fat consumed, but it's a high nutritional price to pay for reducing a serving of potato chips from 150 to 70 calories. If you must have potato chips, you'd be better off cutting back on the fat by buying those that are baked.

## FOOD FOR THOUGHT

- *Consumer Reports* found that a single serving of certain fruits and vegetables grown in the United States can expose children to dangerously high levels of pesticides, which may cause flulike symptoms, and according to the authors, chronic exposure can lead to brain damage. One serving (¾ cup) of winter squash would expose 77 percent of five-year-olds to unsafe levels of pesticides. *All fruits and vegetables should be thoroughly washed or peeled.*
- One Do-Si-Do Girl Scout cookie has 57 calories and 2.67 g of fat, and a serving of four Thin Mint Girl Scout cookies amounts to 140 calories with 70 of those calories coming from fat! So if you thought just because the cookies come from Girl Scouts that they're good for you, you might want to think again.

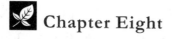 Chapter Eight

# Think Before You Drink— Anything

## 90. Rubbing in the Hard Facts About Alcohol

"Bottoms up!" can be a downer for more people in more ways than they realize.

- Alcohol is not a stimulant, but a sedative and depressant of the central nervous system.
- It can suppress immune system functions, increasing the risk of infection and susceptibility to disease.
- It interferes with proper nutrient absorption.
- It can alter enzymes that normally detoxify carcinogens.
- It is a teratogenic drug. (Pregnant women who drink may endanger their unborn children by causing fetal alcohol syndrome, which can result in low birth weight, brain damage, and physical malformation.)
- It depletes the body of B vitamins (especially folic acid) as well as substantial amounts of calcium, magnesium, zinc, and other trace minerals, all of which are essential emotion energizers.

- It impedes the formation and storage of glycogen in the liver; in other words, it reduces your fitness fuel.
- It impairs coordination and reduces the contractile strength of muscles.
- It worsens allergic reactions to foods.
- It is capable of rupturing veins.
- Its dehydrating properties (which cause morning-after thirst) can destroy brain cells by withdrawing necessary water from them.
- Chronic use can cause memory lapses, impaired learning ability, motor disturbances, and general disorientation.
- Over one million Americans are allergic to ingredients in alcoholic beverages that can cause severe adverse reactions.
- Four drinks a day are capable of causing organ damage.
- Anyone who has acquired a tolerance to alcohol might need larger doses of sedatives or tranquilizers to be effective. This hazardous combination increases the possibility of an unwitting overdose.
- Alcohol can interact adversely with more than one hundred medications, with effects ranging from simple nausea to sudden death.

**CAUTION** Unless you have asked and been told by your physician that you can have a drink with another drug, **DON'T!**

## 91. Beer Is Nothing to Cheer About

It's touted as the ultimate reward for a hard day's work, winning ball games, getting together with friends, and celebrating jobs well done—but that doesn't mean that beer is something to cheer about.

The alcohol in a 12-ounce can of beer is just as intoxicating as the alcohol in a 5-ounce glass of wine; furthermore, beer contains more than just barley, water, malt, hops, and yeast—a lot more.

### BEER ADDITIVES THAT BREW TROUBLE

- *Aspergillus oryzae,* a fungus source suspected of producing a carcinogen during metabolism.

- Papain, shown to be an antigen which, besides causing a specific allergic response, can enlarge ranges of sensitivity.
- Acacia (gum arabic), a foam stabilizer gushing with drawbacks (see section 26).
- Alginate (propylene glycol alginate), which has been shown to cause fetal and maternal deaths in laboratory animals and is considered a health risk for pregnant women.
- Calcium disodium EDTA, which can cause gastrointestinal upsets and kidney damage. (**Note:** EDTA has blood-thinning properties that might affect dosage levels if you are taking anticoagulant medication.)
- Sulfites galore (potassium metabisulfite, sodium bisulfate, sodium hydrosulfite, sodium metabisulfite) used as antioxidants and potentially dangerous for many people. (See section 30.)
- Artificial colors, including FD&C Blue No. 1, Red No. 40, and Yellow No. 5. (See section 86.)
- Nitrosamines (see section 49), unintentionally formed when malted barley is dried by direct firing, but nonetheless carcinogenic. (The U.S. brewing industry has modified its barley-drying process and reduced nitrosamine levels, but nitrosamines at any level are still nitrosamines.)

## 92. The Heavy Truth About Light Beers

No matter how you spell it (light or lite), low-calorie beers aren't weight reducers.

A 12-ounce glass of light beer that should contain approximately 98 calories, or one-third fewer calories than regular beer (approximately 150 calories), sometimes has about as many calories as regular beer. Michelob Light, for example, has 135 calories—only 5 calories less than regular Coors, and only 1 calorie less than Hamm's. And if you are dieting, 50 fewer calories a glass is about as significant as not eating five potato chips—which, if you're a beer drinker, you will probably eat anyway.

Light beers do have less alcohol than regular brews, but not enough to deem them safe for indiscriminate consumption by pregnant women, or anyone with sulfite sensitivity.

## 93. Nonalcoholic Trade-Offs Pay Off

For drinkers who enjoy the taste of malt and hops, but don't want the calories or consequences of alcohol, nonalcoholic beers are probably the best trade-offs around.

Compared with an average of 150 calories in 12 ounces of regular beer, nonalcoholic beer contains about 50 calories. And as far as alcohol goes, you would have to drink about a hundred bottles of nonalcoholic beer on the wall to come close to consuming 6 ounces.

Nonalcoholic beer, by law, can contain only trace amounts of alcohol (½ percent by volume), which is less than what you get in a tablespoon of most over-the-counter cough and cold medicines. (**Note:** Products that are labeled "alcohol free" cannot contain *any* alcohol.)

**CAUTION** Nonalcoholic beer is contraindicated for alcoholics.

## 94. The Grapes of Wrath

Whoever said, *"In vino veritas"* wasn't talking about truth in wine labeling. Despite being one of the most cherished beverages around the world, most people know little more about wine than that it is fermented grape juice (or in the case of sake, a Japanese wine, fermented rice).

Wine lovers will argue that labels tell a lot. They give such important information as where the wine comes from, who produced it, and when and where it was bottled. A label that doesn't give the name of the vineyard where the grapes were grown indicates that the wine may be a blend of wines, usually of inferior taste, since the good wines in a blend are used to upgrade the mediocre ones. A label without a vintage year also indicates a blend of wines from different years. (In California it is legal to add 5 percent of wine from another year to any vintage bottle.) Wine labels will also list the name of the importer and the alcohol content by volume, which can vary from 8.5 percent (a few French and German wines) to 21 percent (sherry and port). American wines generally have an alcohol content of 12 to 14 percent.

But wine labels don't tell you what else you are getting; for example, sulfur dioxide or potassium metabisulfite (which are used to kill bacteria on grapes, or stop yeast action when fermentation has reached the desired point), both of which can seriously endanger sulfite-sensitive individuals (see section 30).

Other chemicals used in wine making that are potential health hazards for many people are:

- Acacia (gum arabic)
- Albumen (egg white)
- Antifoaming and defoaming agents, such as polyoxyethylene-40-monostearate and silicon dioxide
- Casein, potassium salt of casein, and milk powder
- Copper sulfate
- Ferrocyanide compounds
- Lactic and malted acids
- Mineral oil
- Propylene glycol

At this time the government permits wine makers to use over eighty additives. All are certainly not used in any one wine, and many are removed before bottling, but if you have any questions about what's in the wine you are drinking I suggest you write to the wineries. Their addresses are usually on the labels. If not, your local wine merchant can probably get them for you.

## 95. The "French Paradox" Explained

Despite the fact that the French eat a diet of foods extremely high in fat and cholesterol, they have one of the lowest rates of heart disease in the world. Researchers believe this is because of the red wine they drink with meals. Reserveratrol, a member of the polyphenol-flavonoid family that has been shown to reduce the risk of heart disease and stroke by inhibiting the formation of blood clots and LDL (the bad cholesterol), is a compound found in the skin and seeds of grapes. That, along with catechins and anthocyanidin, the antioxidant responsible for the deep purple color of grapes, is believed to account for the "French Paradox."

But you don't have to be a wine drinker to reap the same rewards. Purple grape juice also contains reserveratrol (although in smaller quantities), and supplements are available. I'd suggest taking either one 1,000 mcg reserveratrol capsule daily or two 30 mg polyphenol capsules.

## 96. Why Wine Coolers Are Not So Hot

Wine coolers look like soft drinks, but they are half alcohol (6 percent by volume) and half fruit juice, and contain more sugar than almost any other beverage around.

The majority of brands boast that they're made with "natural" fruit juice, and that they contain "no artificial flavors." But a close look at labels reveals that they contain artificial colors, along with sulfur dioxide, potassium sorbate, and sodium benzoate, all of which can cause a wide variety of allergic reactions (see section 28), and added sugar.

**CAUTION** These are alcoholic beverages and should be kept out of the reach of children, who can easily mistake them for soft drinks. They are also contraindicated for alcoholics, or anyone taking any medications—*particularly* antidepressants, barbiturates, painkillers, and disulfiram (Antabus).

## 97. Liquor Facts That Won't Raise Your Spirits

If you are a drinker, the good news is that 80 to 100 proof whiskeys contain sufficient alcohol (40 to 50 percent) to destroy bacteria, control yeast, and eliminate the need for antifoaming agents. So except for a little ethylenediaminetetraacetate, which is used in brewing, and some questionably safe caramel coloring, most hard liquors are relatively additive free. The bad news is that there are no labels to tell you which ones aren't.

If you're a Scotch drinker, there is more bad news. Because of the way malted barley is dried, Scotch has been found to contain small amounts of carcinogenic nitrosamines. And there's even more bad news if you are into liqueurs or premixed cocktails. These contain artificial colorings, flavorings, and synthetic crème bases. There are some products that use real cream (Bailey's Original Irish Cream Liqueur, for instance), but because of its cost, the cream in many "crème" liqueurs is generally nondairy creamer (see section 65). Check the label before you drink. Alcohol and additives are enough of a nutritional body blow without adding saturated fat.

**NOTE** Real cream liqueurs should be refrigerated after opening to prevent spoilage.

## 98. Taking the Fizz Out of Soft Drinks

Not counting the myriad fruit-flavored beverages such as Kool-Aid, Tang, and Hi-C, 21 percent of the sugar in the American diet comes from soft drinks! That's more than just an unhealthy consumption of empty calories. It is a dangerous overload of caffeine (see section 56) and potentially hazardous, nutrient-depleting additives.

### HARD FACTS ABOUT SOFT DRINKS

- Soft drinks contain large amounts of phosphorus, which can throw off the body's calcium/phosphorus ratio (twice as much calcium as phosphorus), decreasing calcium as well as reducing your body's ability to use it.
- For anyone over age forty, soft drinks can be especially hazardous because the kidneys are less able to excrete excess phosphorus, causing depletion of vital calcium.
- Heavy soft-drink consumption can interfere with your body's metabolization of iron and diminish nerve impulse transmission.
- Sodas may contain—but are not required to disclose—such ingredients as ethyl alcohol and sodium alginate (see section 26).

- Cola drinks can interact adversely with antacids, possibly causing constipation, calcium loss, hypertension, nausea, vomiting, headaches, and kidney damage.
- Soft drinks can decrease the antibacterial action of penicillin and ampicillin.
- The average 12-ounce cola has 150 calories and over an ounce (10 teaspoons) of refined sugar; a 12-ounce 7 UP has 7½ teaspoons of sugar.
- Many diet sodas that are low in calories are *high* in sodium.

**COMMENTS AND CAUTIONS** Salt is just as dangerous to your health as sugar (see section 110), and sometimes causes more upset for dieters, who don't understand that it causes water retention (which can add pounds despite your subtraction of calories).

## 99. The Unwatered-Down Truth About Water

A human being can live for weeks without food, but for only a few days without water. It is our most important nutrient; nothing takes place in our bodies without it.

- It is the best solvent for all the products of digestion.
- It is essential for removing wastes. (People who drink lots of fluids reduce the risk of colon cancer because they are less likely to be constipated, and therefore carcinogen-carrying stool may not linger in the colon.)
- It is indispensable for transporting nutrients, building tissues, and regulating body temperature.
- It has no known toxicity when unadulterated, though an intake of 1½ gallons (16 to 24 glasses) in about an hour could be dangerous to an adult and kill an infant.
- Men who drink six 8-ounce glasses of water per day are about half as likely to get bladder cancer as men who consume less than a glass daily, according to a recent study in the *New England Journal of Medicine*.

- Not all liquids count as water equivalents if you're going for your eight glasses a day. Fruit juice, herb tea, decaffeinated coffee or tea, and fat-free and 1 percent milk do equal 100 percent water. Caffeinated drinks (sodas, iced tea, coffee, black or green tea) equal only 50 percent water. Alcoholic drinks equal 0 percent water.

**CAUTIONS AND COMMENTS** Thirst is not a reliable indicator of water needs, especially in children and the elderly. Extreme temperatures (hot and cold) and exercise increase water loss. Always drink extra fluids on airplanes and in any environment with dry, recirculated air. If your urine is amber instead of pale yellow, you probably need more water.

## 100. How Safe Is Your Tap Water?

Without question, water is the elixir of life—but it may be poisoning millions of us daily. Water contamination is here and it's on the rise. (The Environmental Protection Agency has a priority list of more than one hundred dangerous water pollutants.) Pesticides, hazardous-waste dumps, and industrial dumping of untreated garbage into rivers and landfills, as well as chemical additives used in the treatment of drinking water, are just some of the contributors to the increasing pollution of our drinking water.

How dangerous are these contaminants? Solvent chemicals, such as polychlorinated biphenyls (PCBs) and chloroform, are suspected carcinogens. Others have been found to cause central nervous system disorders and reproductive problems.

Tap water with the wrong pH (due to improper water treatment of acid rain) can dissolve lead from pipes, subjecting young children to lead poisoning, which can cause mental retardation. Actually, 90 percent of U.S. water systems are over one hundred years old and can't handle twenty-first–century contamination and waste. People living in older homes containing lead pipes should definitely have their water analyzed by the local county health department. In fact, even homes with copper plumbing can have lead-soldered joints that might affect tap water.

There is also the problem of new and emerging microscopic viruses and parasites which can infect at much lower doses and are resistant to chlorine—ones such as cryptosporidium (or "crypto"), which can be deadly for the young, elderly, pregnant women, and those with AIDS or on chemotherapy.

**COMMENTS AND CAUTIONS** To find out what's in your municipal tap water, contact your local water department. (Municipal water supplies in all cities are regulated by the Environmental Protection Agency, which requires an annual public statement describing the city's water supply and the quality of its water.) The information is free. Also, be sure to find out how much—or how little—fluoride you're getting. The U.S. Public Health Service recommends 0.7 to 1.2 ppm (parts per million) although the EPA now allows 4 ppm. Most health experts concede that fluoride is beneficial, but too much fluoride has been cited as increasing the risk of bone cancer and hip fractures.

## 101. The Hazards of Home Water Filters

More and more people are being solicited by water filtering companies, which come to your home, test your water, and frighten you enough to sign up for an installation of their product right on the spot.

There are different systems used for processing water that comes from your public supply, and you should be aware of the drawbacks of all of them.

### THE REVERSE-OSMOSIS SYSTEM

Reverse osmosis (RO) has been used for years by industries for large-scale removal of salt from seawater to produce drinking water. Home RO systems remove not only salts, but also sediments and other minerals, cleansing water of chemicals and providing clean, clear taste.

A good reverse-osmosis system will have an NSF (National Sanitation Foundation) seal. Along with the seal, the manufacturer will list the contaminants the system is designed to remove. The good news is that the NSF certificate means that the product does filter what it claims it does, and does not add anything harmful to the water. The bad news is that only half the products on the market are certified. (Look for one that has an "absolute" 1-micron filter, or says that it's "standard 53 for cyst removal.") Noncertified RO systems are not that effective in processing inorganic contaminants, and *should be tested periodically to monitor the performance of the system.* A filter may be able to eliminate the large molecules that add tastes and odors long after it has lost the ability to remove small organic contaminants. And all filters may lose their chemical-removing capacity long before your water flow becomes sluggish.

**CAUTION** A filter can also be loaded with bacteria and not show a reduced flow rate.

## ACTIVATED CARBON FILTERS

These remove undissolved metals such as iron, lead, manganese, and copper, and are best for improving taste and appearance and removing organic chemicals. They can't, however, remove microscopic parasites such as cryptosporidium. They also do not remove magnesium or calcium; water softeners are needed for that.

**CAUTION** Water softeners add sodium to the water, which can unhealthily increase your daily salt intake. Also, activated carbon filters that are not changed on a regular basis can become fouled with harmful contaminants. (Avoid units containing silver as a bacteriostat. Silver has not been shown to be an effective bacteria killer and can be harmful in itself if it leaches into your drinking water.)

## DISTILLERS

These heat water to the boiling point in a chamber. Contaminated liquids remain trapped in the chamber, while other liquids that boil at lower temperatures are vented off as vapors. The steam is then cooled until it condenses into a purified state; then it is collected in a storage reservoir until ready for use.

A distiller is not as effective at removing organic contaminants as it is at removing inorganic dissolved solids, such as lead, salts, and dirt. (Using an activated charcoal filter with a distiller will increase its organic-removal rate to over 90 percent.) Distillers also require electricity for their heating elements, and when in operation they produce a large amount of heat (often enough to heat a small room), which may or may not be desirable, depending on their location and the time of year. At this writing only one product is approved by the NSF.

**CAUTION** A distiller must be descaled regularly. If instructions aren't followed carefully, the processed water can be worse instead of better.

## 102. Hitting the Bottled Alternatives

Just because water is sold in a bottle doesn't mean that it is pure. All water, except distilled, is mineral water and contains impurities (though not necessarily harmful ones).

### MINERAL WATER CONFUSION

Minerals in water are measured by a lump measurement known as "total dissolved solid" (TDS). If a bottled water has 500 ppm (parts per million) or more of TDS, it must be labeled "mineral water," even if the minerals themselves have little to do with the water's quality. On the other hand, if the water has less than 250 ppm it cannot be labeled as mineral water. (Bottled waters with less than 500 ppm must be labeled "low mineral content"; those with TDS above 1,500 must be labeled "high mineral content.")

This has caused confusion for consumers and consternation for bottlers. Perrier just barely made it as a mineral water with 545 ppm TDS. Poland Spring, which has been calling itself a mineral water for more than seventy years, is too pure (less than 126 ppm TDS for both its still and sparkling waters) and had to change its label. And Canada Dry Club Soda had to plead for an exemption to keep its well-recognized label, when it was discovered that the beverage contains 536 ppm TDS. Some bottled "mineral waters" may actually have fewer dissolved minerals than many city water supplies.

"Natural" mineral water, sparkling or still, usually comes from a spring and contains only the minerals present in the water as it flows from the ground.

## TAPPING INTO SPRING WATER

All "spring water" must, under truth-in-labeling laws, come from a spring (Deer Park 100% Spring Water, Evian Natural Spring Water). It may already be carbonated, as is the case with Vittelloise Natural Spring Water, or have carbonation added, which is what Deer Park Sparkling 100% Spring Water does.

The word *natural* implies that the water has not been processed in any way before bottling, whereas plain "spring water" may or may not go right into the bottle. Anything simply labeled "drinking water" generally comes from a well or the tap, and is usually processed before bottling. Bulk waters are generally purified tap water. The word *spring* is often cleverly used as part of a company's name so that it appears to be a description of its product, when it is not.

**COMMENTS AND CAUTIONS**  One out of every five bottled water products is little more than tap water with minor treatment. Check to see that the bottled water comes from a protected underground source, or has been treated by one of the filtration methods mentioned in section 101. If the label does not display this information, look for an 800 number or address on the bottle and ask the company.

## STILL VERSUS SPARKLING

Still water has no gas bubbles. Sparkling water is made bubbly by dissolved carbon dioxide gas, which can occur naturally in subsurface water or be added later. (The gas in most "naturally sparkling" waters, such as Perrier and Saratoga, is drawn off at the spring and reinjected during bottling.)

Still water can be carbonated with either natural carbon dioxide (Poland Spring Sparkling fizzes its Maine water with carbon dioxide mined in Colorado) or manufactured carbon dioxide, which is what Canada Dry Club Soda uses. The difference? Natural carbon dioxide usually produces longer-lasting bubbles.

## CLUB SODA AND SELTZER

If you want carbonated water with no added frills (minerals or mineral salts), go for seltzer. It is filtered, carbonated tap water, period. Club soda is also filtered, carbonated tap water, but minerals and mineral salts are frequently added. If you are trying to cut down on your sodium, choose seltzer. Six ounces of Schweppes Club Soda have 26 mg of salt.

## 103. Any Questions About Chapter 8?

*A landfill has just been built about a mile from my home, and I am worried about my well water being contaminated. A company in my area tests water, but I've heard that it tells everyone something is wrong with the water just to sell its purifiers. Can I test my own water?*

If you want the whole truth and nothing but, you want a certified lab to test your drinking water. The EPA has a Safe Drinking Water Hotline and it will give you the name of a state-approved testing lab and provide you with a copy of the EPA guidelines. Fees are around $15 to $20 and well worth it. Meanwhile, until you are sure that your water is safe, you should take the following emergency measures:

- Let your water run three to four minutes every day before using it. This will help flush out any lead, calcium, and cobalt that may be lodging in your pipes.
- Boil your water (uncovered) for at least twenty minutes before using it. Boiling can kill bacteria and remove some organic chemicals. (But boiling will *not* remove chemical additives, metals, or other contaminants.)

- If you are worried about trihalomethanes, whip your water in a blender for fifteen minutes with the top off. Aeration removes chlorine and chlorinated organics.

**CAUTION**  If you suspect that chlorinated solvents or pesticides are in your water, be aware that these chemicals can be absorbed through the skin and are volatile. *Taking one fifteen-minute shower can be as toxic as drinking eight glasses of contaminated water.*

### *Why is it that some alcoholic drinks give me a hangover while others don't?*

Distilled spirits have varying amounts of substances known as congeners (pronounced *con-jen-ers*). They are the impurities that form during the fermentation and maturation of liquor, as well as contribute to its flavor. They also cause hangover. Though alcohol can be eliminated fairly rapidly from the body, congeners cannot.

There are different types and amounts of congeners in drinks, and their adverse effects depend on your sensitivity to them. Some people can knock back six shots of vodka without blinking an eye, but give them a jigger of bourbon and they are looped. For others, it could be just the opposite.

Generally, the more congeners a beverage has, the more splitting the hangover. Bourbon has the most congeners; gin and vodka have the fewest (especially those, such as Skyy Vodka, which use controlled distillation methods that eliminate specific impurities). Brandy seems to produce the majority of hangovers, followed in morning-after infamy by red wine (which has substances very similar to congeners), rum, whiskey, white wine, gin, and vodka.

## FOOD FOR THOUGHT

- The *American Journal of Clinical Nutrition* has reported that, compared with juice or water, having one alcoholic drink before a

meal led to eating 200 extra calories—on top of the added calories in the drink itself.

- Nearly 90 percent of all violations of the Safe Drinking Water
  Act are not reported in the government database that alerts consumers and triggers legal action when water systems don't meet
  health standards.
- Oxygen-enriched waters are said to be enhanced with up to forty
  times the normal oxygen concentration found naturally in water.
  They claim to boost energy by increasing oxygen saturation of
  the red blood cells. To date, though, there is no published medical
  evidence to validate such claims.

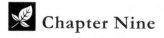 Chapter Nine

# For Whom the Dinner Bell Tolls

### 104. The Big Supper Mistake

For most people, dinner is the largest meal of the day, and it shouldn't be. This is the time when we need the least number of calories, yet consume the most. It's the time when we consume the greatest amount of protein, fat, carbohydrates, and sodium, but need them the least. It's the meal we feel makes up for skipped breakfasts and poor lunches, but it doesn't. It's the most misunderstood, mishandled meal of the day.

Before sitting down for dinner it is important to consider what else you've eaten that day. Ignoring the fact that you had a croissant for breakfast and a hamburger with fries for lunch can be risky if you're planning to have a full-course steak meal. Dinner can take you well over your recommended daily limit of fat, protein, sodium, and calories, and trip you up in innumerable nutritional ways. The following guide has been designed to help prevent this from happening.

## HEALTHY AMOUNTS FOR HEALTHIER LIVING

### Calories and Fat

| AGE | RECOMMENDED DAILY CALORIE INTAKE | RECOMMENDED DAILY FAT INTAKE | |
|---|---|---|---|
| (CHILDREN) | | | |
| 1–3 | 1,300 | 8 tsp. | 35.2 g |
| 4–6 | 1,700 | 11 tsp. | 48.4 g |
| 7–10 | 2,400 | 15 tsp. | 66.0 g |
| (MALES) | | | |
| 11–14 | 2,700 | 17 tsp. | 74.8 g |
| 15–18 | 2,800 | 18 tsp. | 79.2 g |
| 19–22 | 2,900 | 18 tsp. | 79.2 g |
| 23–50 | 2,700 | 17 tsp. | 74.8 g |
| 51–74 | 2,400 | 15 tsp. | 66.0 g |
| 75+ | 2,050 | 13 tsp. | 57.2 g |
| (FEMALES) | | | |
| 11–14 | 2,220 | 14 tsp. | 61.6 g |
| 15–22 | 2,100 | 13 tsp. | 57.2 g |
| 23–50 | 2,000 | 13 tsp. | 57.2 g |
| 51–74 | 1,800 | 11 tsp. | 48.4 g |
| 75+ | 1,600 | 11 tsp. | 48.4 g |

### Protein and Sodium

| AGE | RECOMMENDED DAILY PROTEIN INTAKE | RECOMMENDED DAILY SODIUM INTAKE |
|---|---|---|
| (CHILDREN) | | |
| 1–3 | 23 g | 650 mg |
| 4–6 | 30 g | 900 mg |
| 7–10 | 34 g | 1,200 mg |

| AGE | RECOMMENDED DAILY PROTEIN INTAKE | RECOMMENDED DAILY SODIUM INTAKE |
|---|---|---|
| (MALES) | | |
| 11–14 | 45 g | 1,800 mg |
| 15–18 | 56 g | 1,800 mg |
| 19–74+ | 56 g | 2,220 mg |
| | | |
| (FEMALES) | | |
| 11–18 | 46 g | 1,800 mg |
| 19–74+ | 44 g | 2,200 mg |

## 105. Meaty Problems

We eat too much meat for our own good. Just ½ a pound of lean ground beef supplies a woman's entire daily requirement for protein; ¾ of a pound has more than what is recommended for a man.

There is no question that meat is an excellent source of protein and that protein is the major source of building material for the body, but eating too much of it can be hazardous to your health (see section 107) and eating too much in the form of animal flesh can be even more hazardous. Aside from meat's potential for supplying us with more protein than we need and more saturated fat than we should have, it is insidiously supplying us with drugs we don't want. The majority of American livestock is routinely given subtherapeutic doses of antibiotics such as penicillin and tetracycline. Because subtherapeutic doses are smaller than those needed to control an actual infection, they

The Union of Concerned Scientists recently estimated that 24.6 million pounds of antibiotics, about 70 percent of total U.S. antibiotic production, are fed to chickens, pigs, and cows for nontherapeutic purposes.

kill off susceptible bacteria and allow resistant ones to thrive, promoting the spread of antibiotic-resistant bacteria—which is being transmitted to humans!

The alarming increase of antibiotic-resistant bacteria in humans has caused numerous outbreaks of gastrointestinal infections, as well as dozens of documented cases of antibiotic-resistant salmonellosis (several fatal) caused by the consumption of hamburger from cattle that had been treated with chlortetracycline as a growth promoter.

The presence of these drug residues poses enormous health risks for everyone.

- A person allergic to penicillin, for instance, could suffer the same adverse reaction by eating a roast beef sandwich if the animal the beef came from had been dosed with that drug.
- Antibiotics that have been used successfully to treat numerous illnesses and infections are being rendered ineffective because of our increasing acquisition of antibiotic-resistant bacteria. (Already, 20 percent of the organisms responsible for strep throat can no longer be killed by tetracycline.)
- Many chemicals being used (albeit illegally) in animal feed are known carcinogens.

Unfortunately, there is no way to tell if your meat (or chicken, eggs, or milk) is tainted with drug residues, but you can minimize the risk to yourself and your family in several ways.

- Eat fewer animal products.
- Eat leaner animal products.
- Eat your steaks and burgers well done.
- Buy organic meat (free of hormones and antibiotics).

**COMMENTS AND CAUTIONS** Be aware that animal products also contain dioxin and its chemical cousins, the furans and PCBs (polychlorinated biphenyls), toxic carcinogens that can alter DNA and lead to any number of birth defects and diseases. These dioxin toxins are released into the atmosphere mainly through emissions from incinerators. They make their way from the air, water, soil, and sediment into plants. Animals eat the plants and people eat the animals, a scary food cycle. Because dioxin and its fat-soluble cousins reside in fat, the importance of minimizing your consumption of animal fat cannot be overstated!

## 106. Mad Cow Disease

So far American cows have tested free of mad cow disease, or bovine spongiform encephalopathy (BSE), which has killed nearly 200,000 British and European cattle. The human variant, Creutzfeldt-Jakob disease (CJD), contracted by eating meat from an infected animal, has already claimed more than one hundred lives. No one knows how widespread the contamination of beef is, but remains of BSE-infected cows were shipped all over the world as beef by-products for cattle feed and reached more than eighty countries. American officials banned British cattle feed in 1988, as soon as scientists implicated it in BSE, and later barred the use of products from domestic cows as well.

Just the facts:

- You can't contract CJD unless you eat meat from an infected animal.
- Chicken and pigs are unlikely to have mad cow disease.
- The greatest dangers come from burgers, sausages, and meat still attached to the bone (such as a T-bone steak). These products may contain nerve fibers, which means they're more likely to contain the prions (infectious proteins) involved. (If you can't resist eating steak, flank steak and filet mignon are presumably safer.)

## 107. Resolving the Protein Predicament

Everyone knows that protein is essential for life. It is vital for the growth, development, and repair of all body tissues; regulation of the body's water balance; the formation of hormones and enzymes necessary for basic life functions and antibodies needed to fight infection; and more. But too much of a good thing can be bad for you.

## THE PROBLEMS OF TOO MUCH PROTEIN

- It can shorten life expectancy.
- It can increase the risk of cancer and heart disease.
- It can stress and damage the liver and kidneys.
- It can deplete calcium from bones and promote osteoporosis.
- It can cause fluid imbalance and dehydration.
- It can be hazardous to premature infants.
- It can contribute significantly to obesity.
- It increases your need for vitamin $B_6$.

Excessive protein consumption is generally the result of diets over-loaded with meat, cheese, poultry, eggs, and fish, and undersupplied with legumes, grains, and vegetables.

Meat, cheese, poultry, eggs, and fish are *complete proteins*. They provide the proper balance of all the essential amino acids (those that cannot, like others, be manufactured by the human body and must be obtained from food or supplements), and are widely—but erroneously—believed to be (a) healthier, (b) nonfattening, and (c) harmless when eaten in large amounts.

Legumes, grains, and vegetables are *incomplete proteins*. They lack certain essential amino acids and are not used efficiently when eaten alone, which might account for their being widely—but erroneously—believed to be (a) optional, (b) fattening, and (c) wholesome when eaten in small amounts.

## PUTTING PROTEIN IN PERSPECTIVE

- Complete proteins generally have more fat than incomplete proteins.
- Incomplete proteins combined with rice, corn, or grains can become wholesome, low-fat complete proteins.
- *Mixing complete and incomplete proteins can give you better nutrition than having either one alone!*

## 108. Why Not a Low-Fat Chicken in Every Pot?

The same poultry industry that adulterated feed to breed chickens bigger, fatter, and faster is now feeding its birds low-calorie, high-protein food (ingredients unknown) to reduce their fat and increase their price. The result is chickens that have approximately 14 to 21 percent less fat than before.

Everyone knows that less fat is better. What they don't know is that as impressive as a 14 to 21 percent reduction sounds, it's less than 2 g of fat for an average serving of 4 to 6 ounces, which is the amount of fat in half a pat (½ teaspoon) of butter—not very impressive. What makes it even less impressive is that fat reductions vary enormously from brand to brand, and have been found to be even wider within a particular brand.

Chicken has always been lower in fat and cholesterol than red meat, and the major component of its taste is bound in its fat. As long as low-fat chickens have erratic and dubious fat reductions, you're better off defatting your own.

For whole roasters or broilers: Remove the yellow fat globules that are just inside the cavity near the tail. (They can usually be pulled out with your fingers, but a paring knife will ensure success.)

For chicken parts: Yellow fat globules are visible on the thighs and rib cage. Pull or cut them off.

For significant fat reduction: Remove fat *and skin* before cooking. Skinned chicken should be cooked slowly to prevent unappetizing dryness. Braising in a covered pan with water or broth and vegetables is the best way to retain flavor and nutrients.

When making chicken soup, you can leave the skin on while cooking (for flavor), but be sure to skim the fat off when the soup is cool. (**Note:** Capons and large hens have more fat than roasters or broilers.)

**COMMENTS AND CAUTIONS** For years the USDA has allowed poultry processors to dump chicken carcasses into tubs of water to chill them. In the process, the birds gain up to 8 percent of their body weight in water. Consumers then pay chicken prices for water. But, more important, these chickens have been found to be more often contaminated and likely to cause food poisoning. Studies have shown that chickens leave the water baths more contaminated than when they entered. Look for organic, free-range chicken, preferably locally raised and slaughtered.

## 109. The Soy Alternative

For centuries, the Chinese and Japanese have been eating a diet high in soy foods and reaping impressive longevity benefits as well as much lower rates of death from cancer and heart disease than Americans. Soy is one of the few plant foods that is a complete protein containing the proper balance of the eight essential amino acids. The U.S. government recognizes it as a protein alternative equivalent to meat, and, according to the *American Journal of Clinical Nutrition,* "except for premature infants, soy protein can serve as a sole protein source in the human body." As with other vegetable proteins, eating it with a grain such as rice or pasta enhances its nutritional value.

### SOY ADVANTAGES OVER ANIMAL PROTEIN

- Lower in fat
- No cholesterol
- High in phytochemicals
- Good source of fiber
- Good source of minerals such as calcium, iron, magnesium, phosphorus, and the B vitamins thiamin, riboflavin, and niacin

(**Note:** Soybeans—with the exception of tempeh, a fermented whole soybean product—are a poor source of vitamin $B_{12}$. Vegetarians should take supplementary vitamin $B_{12}$.)

### POTENTIAL BENEFITS OF SOY

- Can help lower cholesterol levels.
- Antioxidants present in soy foods may protect against many forms of cancer as well as premature aging.

- Isoflavones in soy may retard bone loss almost as effectively as supplemental estrogen, helping to prevent osteoporosis.
- May slow down or prevent kidney damage in people with impaired kidney function.
- Aids in boosting the immune system.
- May alleviate hot flashes in menopausal women.

## POSSIBLE HEALTH RISKS OF SOY

- Eating huge amounts of soy foods may interfere with thyroid function, triggering goiter (enlargement of the thyroid) and hypothyroidism.

**COMMENTS AND CAUTIONS** There has been some controversy over the high content of phytates in soybeans. Phytates bind to essential minerals such as calcium, iron, and zinc in the digestive tract and prevent them from being absorbed. Soaking and fermenting—as used in making miso, natto, shoyu, tamari, and tempeh (but not tofu, soy milk, texturized soy protein, or soy protein isolate)—significantly reduce the phytate content. But a high phytate content might not be a bad thing. Phytates have been shown in some animal studies to stop the growth of cancerous tumors by binding with the minerals that may feed them. Also, keep in mind that the more processed the soybeans, the less amount of usable soy isoflavones you're getting. (Soy sauce and soy oil have no nutritional value.)

## 110. Please Pass on the Salt

You know those two shakers that are on dinner tables? Stay away from the one with the small holes: It's a killer. Asking someone to pass it to you is committing nutritional hara-kiri. High salt consumption can cause hypertension, migraine headaches, abnormal fluid retention, and potassium loss; interfere with proper utilization of protein; and increase your chances of heart disease and other ailments.

Sodium is in virtually all our foods. The average American consumes about a bowling ball of it (15 pounds) each year. So, if you think you don't eat much salt because you never eat pretzels or chips, you had better think again before dinner.

## SNEAKY SUPPER SALT TRAPS

- Tomato juice is a great low-calorie appetizer, but it is high in sodium. Six ounces of Del Monte's has 478 mg; Campbell's has 555 mg.
- Condiments look harmless, but one 11-calorie dill pickle has 1,426 mg of sodium.
- Use 2 tablespoons of ketchup on (or in) your meatloaf and you have added 308 mg of sodium; 2 tablespoons of mustard will give you 444 mg.
- If you are starting with soup, a cup of regular chicken noodle has 979 mg; a cup of onion has 1,051 mg.
- Add a cup of raw celery to your salad and you have 151 mg of sodium; add 2 tablespoons of Italian dressing and you have 624 mg more.
- Eat a 2-inch square of cornbread with your meal and you have piled on another 283 mg.
- A 1-pound lobster has 1,359 mg, and that's without the melted butter, which has 1,120 mg in a half cup.
- If you want cooked carrots, you'll get only 51 mg in a cup if they are fresh; if they are canned, you'll get 366 mg.
- A standard piece of apple pie for dessert has 486 mg; black coffee, 59 mg.

Put them all together and they spell trouble, with a capital T.

**MINDELL HEALTH MORSEL** If you need to add salt while cooking, add it at the end and you'll need less. The longer food cooks, the more the salty flavor is muted and at the end, the final taste is on the top layer.

## 111. Are You Getting the Full Fish Story?

We have all been told that we should eat more fish—and there are lots of good reasons to do so (see section 112)—but there's a lot we have *not* been told about some of the fish we're already eating.

## CATCH-OF-THE-DAY CAUTIONS

While the FDA and the EPA argue over what are "safe" levels of mercury in fish, this is a fast look at those fish you might want to keep off your plate permanently, and those you should only eat limited quantities of each month.

### Avoid If Pregnant

Shark, swordfish, king mackerel, tilefish, tuna steaks, sea bass, marlin, halibut, walleye, largemouth bass

(Methylmercury can cause damage to the nervous system of an unborn child. Large fish that feed on other fish accumulate the highest amount of methylmercury and pose the greatest risk to people who eat them regularly. These fish are also not recommended for nursing mothers, young children, and the elderly.)

### Safer Fish Trade-Offs

Trout (farmed), catfish (farmed), salmon (farmed), shrimp, Mrs. Paul's (farm-raised) fish sticks

**COMMENTS AND CAUTIONS** If you're pregnant, you can eat a variety of other fish. Keep portions between 3 to 6 ounces and within an average of no more than 12 ounces of cooked fish a week. If you have questions about mercury levels in any fresh-caught fish, you can call toll-free 1-888-SAFEFOOD. This is the U.S. Food and Drug Administration, Center for Food Safety and Applied Nutrition, Food Information Hotline. (Or go to www.cfsan.fda.gov.)

## 112. Yes, You Still Should Have Fish for Dinner

Fish offers enough substantial health benefits for the American Medical Association, the *Journal of the National Cancer Institute,* and virtually all nutritionists to recommend eating it two to four times weekly. The reason: omega-3 fatty acids (FA). EPA (eicosapentaenoic acid) and DHA (docosahexaenoic acid) are the two fatty acids in this group that have been found to have potentially remarkable preventive and curative properties.

## BENEFITS OF OMEGA-3 FATTY ACIDS

- Can reduce harmful cholesterol and triglycerides, and lower the risk of heart attack or stroke.
- Can help to prevent fatal heart rhythm disturbances.
- Can reduce the "stickiness" of blood platelet cells and the amount of fibrin in the blood, reducing the risk of clot formation.
- Help reduce pain and inflammation of rheumatoid arthritis.
- Provide relief from the itching and scaling of psoriasis.
- Reduce the body's rejection of tissue grafts.
- Aid in the reduction and severity of migraine headaches.
- Fight harmful effects of prostaglandins (which lower immunity and encourage tumor growth) and help prevent breast cancer.
- Help in preventing arteriosclerosis.

## BEST FISH SOURCES OF OMEGA-3s

| FISH | GRAMS PER 3½-OUNCE SERVING |
| --- | --- |
| Norway sardines | 5.1 |
| Chinook salmon | 3.04 |
| Atlantic markerel | 2.18 |
| Pink salmon | 1.87 |
| Canned light albacore tuna | 1.69 |
| Sablefish | 1.39 |
| Atlantic herring | 1.09 |
| Rainbow trout (U.S.) | 1.08 |
| Pacific oyster | 0.84 |
| Striped bass | 0.64 |
| Channel catfish | 0.61 |
| Ocean perch | 0.51 |

| FISH | GRAMS PER 3½-OUNCE SERVING |
| --- | --- |
| Blue crab (cooked, canned) | 0.46 |
| Pacific halibut | 0.45 |
| Shrimp | 0.39 |
| Yellowtail flounder | 0.30 |

If you don't like fish or cannot eat it on a regular basis, fish oil supplements are an alternative. Ten capsules of concentrated marine lipids usually supply 1.8 g of EPA. (A 4-ounce serving of salmon contains about 1 g.) Cod-liver oil contains EPA, too, but amounts vary according to brand, and it hasn't been shown to be effective in lowering blood cholesterol. Also, cod-liver oil has high levels of vitamins A and D, which can be toxic in large amounts.

**CAUTION** Taking large doses of omega-3 supplements may cause excessive bruising and bleeding after minor trauma in some individuals. Anyone with a tendency to such bruising and bleeding is advised to avoid these supplements entirely. As with large doses of vitamin E, this could result in internal bleeding. Check with your doctor before starting on omega-3 or any other supplement regimen.

## 113. Pasta Pitfalls

Pasta is the complex carbohydrate muscle fuel that athletes load up on before competitions and the preferred food for diabetics because it doesn't cause rapid blood sugar rise after eating. But pastas are made from different types of flour, and different flours come from different grains, and different grains have different benefits and risks for different people (see section 129).

Perhaps the most common pasta pitfall is the most common pasta: spaghetti. Many commercial brands are not made with durum wheat, which is used to make durum flour and semolina and contains more protein than ordinary enriched pasta. Also, manufacturers tend to recommend cooking their products longer than necessary, which increases calories, depletes nutrients, and renders pasta more starchy and less desirable for use by diabetics. (When overcooked, pasta's sugars enter the bloodstream faster, causing insulin to overreact and bring blood sugar down, resulting in fatigue and hunger.) Pasta should be cooked *al dente*—that is, firm and slightly chewy.

Pasta packed in clear cellophane, or with large cellophane windows, is subject to nutrient loss. And any pasta containing disodium phosphate (which is added to make it quick cooking) should be avoided.

Still another pasta pitfall is the tendency to smother it with rich, creamy sauces that are mostly fat. This can not only harm your arteries and pile on the pounds, but diminish alertness. Because fat is hard to digest, blood is waylaid in the stomach for hours instead of energizing the brain. (*Tip:* Sprinkling pasta with a bit of olive oil, which has been found to be a cholesterol-lowering fat, and adding some cooked clams or mussels can turn it into a really wholesome dinner.) Eating pasta without protein can leave you feeling sluggish an hour or two later, so it's advisable to have some sort of protein for an appetizer if you are not going to add it to the pasta itself.

> The greatest pasta pitfall of all is portion size. A portion of pasta is not a platter—it's a cup. And a cup of pasta is about the size of a tennis ball!

There are two general types of pasta: one includes spaghetti, macaroni, shells, and lasagna; the other is noodles, which by law must contain at least 5½ percent egg solids. These add cholesterol and might not be advisable for individuals on a low-cholesterol diet. With the exception of oriental egg noodles, though, Asian noodles are *not* made with eggs. Since they look like noodles but cannot be labeled as such, they are usually marked "imitation noodles" or "alimentary paste" on packages.

If you have gluten intolerance, you should avoid pasta made with wheat. This might sound difficult, but it isn't. Buckwheat pasta is gluten free and can be obtained in health food stores, as can wheatless corn pasta. There are also Chinese bean threads and cellophane noodles (made from mung beans, the cellophane noodles sometimes from seaweed); and Japanese shirataki (also made from mung beans, but with yams and other root plants that are used, too, for Japanese saifun).

**CAUTION** Dried seasonings that are often sold for use with oriental noodles to make soup generally contain MSG.

## 114. Any Questions About Chapter 9?

*I've read all the bad news about grilling steaks, about how barbecuing can produce cancer-causing compounds. Is there any way to avoid this?*
There's no way to avoid it, but if you really love grilled beef you can minimize the carcinogens you get by marinating the steaks before grilling. Researchers who marinated beef in Hawaiian teriyaki and Indian turmeric–garlic marinades found they could reduce carcinogens by as much as 67 percent. According to *Time* magazine, the meat was marinated overnight, but just an hour or two may suffice. Also, according to the *Journal of the National Cancer Institute,* burgers turned every minute while being cooked had 75 to 95 percent fewer total carcinogens than burgers turned only once after five minutes of cooking.

*Every time my mother tells me that I am going to get sick if I keep eating at sushi bars all the time, I wind up having to scream that she's wrong, but don't know how to prove it. Do you have any suggestions?*
First of all, I would suggest you stop screaming at your mother, particularly since she is not wrong. If you are eating a steady diet of raw fish, you're depleting your body of thiamin (vitamin $B_1$), which is known for its beneficial effects on the nervous system and mental attitude. Your screaming might be an indication that you are low on that vitamin already.
All raw fish and shellfish contain a substance that destroys $B_1$, but eating a varied diet makes up for this. Sushi and sashimi are fine sources of nutrients and omega-3 fatty acids, providing the fish is fresh and from uncontaminated waters, but I don't recommend eating them to the exclusion of other foods. If you are eating out that often, try some Italian pastas, or some Mexican rice and bean dishes for variety. They're nutritious,

low in fat, can replace your lost B vitamins—and make your mother happy, too.

*I'm sixty years old and my daughter told me that I should stop eating meat and cheese because it is weakening my bones. I thought protein builds bones. What's the truth?*

While it's true that a diet deficient in protein weakens bones in later life, it is equally true that a high protein intake can increase calcium loss and bone fractures in older women. There are about 350,000 hip fractures each year in the United States and researchers now believe that protein-rich animal foods load the blood with acid, which the body may neutralize by stealing minerals from bone. Our kidneys ordinarily regulate the acidity of our blood by dumping excess acid in the urine, but too much protein can overload them.

Calcium-rich foods help, but a growing number of doctors and nutritionists (myself included) believe that fruits and vegetables may offer the best assistance because they produce acid-neutralizing bases. I'd suggest subtracting some of the animal protein from your diet and start adding portions of broccoli, oranges, tomatoes, and spinach to your daily fare.

## FOOD FOR THOUGHT

- According to the most recent government figures, seafood was to blame for 4.4 percent of all known cases of food-borne illness with an identifiable cause; shellfish was responsible for nearly three-quarters of these seafood-related cases.
- One in eight samples of tuna that was bought in supermarkets and tested by *Consumer Reports* had unacceptable levels of histamine, an odorless, nearly tasteless decomposition chemical that can cause hives and other reactions. And six of eleven samples of "red snapper" were actually other species of fish.

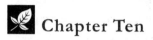 Chapter Ten

# The Hazards of "Health" and Healthy Foods

## 115. All That's Fiber Isn't Fabulous

The American Cancer Institute recommends you eat 25 to 30 g of fiber daily; the average American eats about 15 g. Unfortunately, the average American doesn't know that:

- All fiber is not the same.
- Different fibers have different effects on the body.
- No one type should be eaten to the exclusion of the others.
- Everybody doesn't need the same type or amount of fiber in his or her diet.
- Even the best sources of fiber have nutritional hazards.
- Without a sufficient intake of liquids (six to eight glasses daily), fiber can be constipating.
- Large increases in fiber can be dangerous for individuals with possible nutrient deficiencies (teenagers, the elderly, anyone with an illness or existing medical problem) *and should not be made without first consulting a physician!*

## 116. Know Your Fiber Before You Eat It

### CELLULOSE AND HEMICELLULOSES

These absorb water and facilitate smooth functioning of the large bowel. They "bulk" waste and help move it through the colon rapidly. This not only can prevent constipation, but may also protect against diverticulosis, spastic colon, hemorrhoids, colon cancer, and varicose veins.

Best cellulose sources are whole-wheat flour, bran, cabbage, young peas, green beans, wax beans, broccoli, brussels sprouts, cucumber skins, peppers, apples, and carrots. (These provide insoluble fiber.)

Best hemicellulose sources are bran, cereals, whole grains, brussels sprouts, mustard greens, and beets. (These provide insoluble and soluble fiber.)

**CAUTION** Too much fiber in your diet can cause gas, bloating, nausea, vomiting, and diarrhea, and possibly interfere with the body's ability to absorb protein, as well as such necessary minerals as zinc, calcium, iron, magnesium, and vitamin $B_{12}$. Increased fiber may be contraindicated in certain bowel disorders.

### GUMS AND PECTIN

Gums and pectin primarily influence absorption in the stomach and small bowel. By binding with bile acids, they decrease fat absorption and lower cholesterol levels. They delay stomach emptying by coating the lining of the gut, and slow sugar absorption after a meal, which is helpful to diabetics since it reduces the amount of insulin needed at any one time.

Best sources are oatmeal and other rolled oat products, dried beans, apples, citrus fruits, carrots, cauliflower, cabbage, dried peas, green beans, potatoes, squash, and strawberries.

**CAUTION** Same as for cellulose and hemicellulose, but these can also interfere with the effectiveness of certain antifungal medications containing griseofulvin, such as Grifulvin V, Grisactin, and Fulvicin, which are used to combat fungus infections.

## LIGNIN

Lignin is an insoluble fiber that reduces the digestibility of other fibers. It also binds with bile acids to lower cholesterol and helps speed food through the gut, and can aid in weight loss by providing a feeling of fullness.

Best sources of this type of fiber are found in breakfast cereals, bran, older vegetables (when vegetables age, their lignin content rises and they become less digestible), eggplant, green beans, strawberries, pears, and radishes.

**CAUTIONS** Same as those for other fiber. Also, keep in mind that bran, though a good source of lignin fiber, is mostly cellulose, which does *not* have the cholesterol-lowering properties of pectin and gums.

## 117. Dangers in Natural Foods

Just because something is natural and edible doesn't mean it is good for you, or that it can be consumed indiscriminately. All foods are essentially chemical compounds and affect the way your body functions.

- Natural toxins are present in some of our most wholesome foods.
- Some of our most wholesome foods can destroy some of our most vital nutrients.
- Some of our most vital nutrients can interact adversely with each other and harm us!

In short, the more limited your diet, the more extensively you can jeopardize your health.

## 118. Healthy but Hazardous

### BEEF LIVER

Beef liver is one of the richest sources of natural vitamin A, but vitamin A can be a killer if consumed in excess. Symptoms of toxicity include hair loss, nausea, vomiting, diarrhea, scaly skin, blurred vision, rashes, bone pain, irregular menses, fatigue, headaches, pressure within the skull, and liver enlargement. Excessive consumption of liver by adults (more than half a pound daily, or 4 pounds weekly, for many months) has been linked to a painful brain disorder known as pseudotumor cerebri (PTC), and daily ingestion of as little as 4 ounces can produce toxic effects in infants. Liver is also high in cholesterol, and, because it's the detoxifying organ of the body, may contain high levels of DDT and other hazardous chemicals.

## POTATOES

Potatoes are great complex carbohydrates—no-fat, nutritious suppliers of high-quality vegetable protein, vitamins (especially C), minerals, and other essential nutrients. But when potato skins turn a greenish color (because of chlorophyll buildup), they have accumulated a dangerous chemical called solanine. Solanine, present in and around these green patches, and in eyes that have sprouted, can interfere with the transmission of nerve impulses, and cause jaundice, abdominal pain, vomiting, and diarrhea.

There is controversy about whether solanine is destroyed by cooking, and as long as there is doubt I wouldn't count on it. If you find that your potatoes turn green in storage or sprout eyes, remove the skin and cut away the layer of potato just under it before cooking. (Storing potatoes in paper bags and away from light will inhibit the buildup of solanine.)

There is also controversy among rheumatologists and nutritionists about whether solanine poses a particular hazard for people with arthritis and other joint diseases. Until it is resolved, I'd suggest you assume that it does and be particularly careful about the potatoes you eat if you are afflicted with any of these ailments.

What there is too little controversy about is the amount of pesticides being used on potatoes. In USDA tests done on 694 potato samples, residues of 24 different toxic and carcinogenic pesticides were found. And residues of the equally dangerous postharvest growth inhibitors that are used on potatoes when they go to market remain in the spud itself!

## NUTS AND GRAINS

These are healthy, high-protein sources of B vitamins, fiber, and energy, provided they are free of aflatoxins. Aflatoxins are the by-products of molds that grow on grains and nuts, and may be carcinogenic. (Studies have shown correlations between aflatoxin consumption from foods and increased incidences of liver cancer.)

Aflatoxin levels in susceptible foods (peanuts, for instance) are monitored by the government, but government monitoring often leaves much to be desired—namely, safety. Since cooking doesn't destroy aflatoxins, it is advisable to check nuts and grains before purchasing them (and definitely before eating them) to be sure they are not moldy, shriveled, or discolored. Buy organic whenever possible.

## GRAPEFRUIT JUICE

A great source of vitamin C, vitamins, and fiber, grapefruits also contain lycopene, an antioxidant that protects against heart disease and cancer. But grapefruit juice utilizes the same liver "pathway" as some drugs—which, if taken at the same time, may increase or decrease the effects of these drugs. (Blood pressure medications, antihistamines, cholesterol-lowering drugs, and some antidepressants are among the most commonly affected. Check with your pharmacist.)

## MUSHROOMS

Mushrooms are no-fat, low-sodium, tasty sources of niacin, potassium, and selenium, and great for dieters and cholesterol watchers, provided you don't go out and pick them in the wild. Even the most experienced wild mushroom eaters have been known to make mistakes that have caused them a variety of unpleasant symptoms (nausea, vomiting, cramps, and diarrhea), and in some cases, even death. There is no foolproof way to determine the safety of a wild mushroom, and since the toxic effects of many varieties are either unknown or untreatable, it's best

**177**

to buy mushrooms at your local produce market, provided they have not been treated with a bisulfite solution (see section 30).

## ALFALFA SPROUTS

These sprouted seeds are terrific sources of vitamins C and K, minerals, and numerous micronutrients (often more than contained in the full-grown plant). Low in calories and high in fiber, they are a definite plus in salads—*but only if they are organically grown!* The FDA has advised even healthy adults, not just children or the elderly, to stop eating raw alfalfa, clover, and radish sprouts to avoid getting sick from food poisoning. Raw sprouts are frequently contaminated with salmonella or *E. coli* bacteria. Consumers are urged to ask restaurants to omit them from dishes or to cook them to a high temperature to kill the bacteria.

Additionally, research has shown that overconsumption of alfalfa sprouts can cause an autoimmune form of anemia similar to SLE (systemic lupus erythematosus). The disease is apparently caused by a substance in the sprout that mistakenly becomes part of human protein and sets off an immunological attack against the body.

**CAUTION** Anyone suffering from lupus is advised not to eat any sprouts at all.

## SPINACH
### (Swiss chard, sorrel, parsley, beet greens, rhubarb)

What could possibly be naturally hazardous about Popeye's favorite food and such deep green and leafy others? The answer is oxalic acid, a natural ingredient in these nutrient-rich vegetables and fruits (as well as chocolate) that can inhibit the absorption of their calcium and iron, and bind with calcium to make another insoluble compound that may form kidney or gallbladder stones.

Calcium-rich alternatives *without* absorption-inhibiting oxalic acid are kale, broccoli, and collard greens, which, by the way, are also fine suppliers of B vitamins.

**178**

**CAUTION** Green leafy vegetables are loaded with vitamin C, folate, and other essential nutrients. But they are also rich in vitamin K, which is involved in blood clotting. So if you're taking a blood-thinning medication such as Coumadin (warfarin), eat consistent amounts of these foods (the same amount all the time). Eating more—or a lot less—than usual can alter the effects of these drugs and promote abnormal clotting.

## WHOLE-GRAIN BRAN

Even the king of fiber has a potential health hazard: phytic acid. Like oxalic acid, phytic acid can block absorption of calcium and other minerals from the grain, particularly zinc. Since medical findings seem to indicate that zinc may be required in the synthesis of DNA (the body-as-computer life chip containing all inherited traits and directing all cell activity), anything that diminishes its intake should be considered hazardous.

If you eat a lot of whole-grain cereals with milk, be sure to increase your intake of zinc through other foods. (See section 145.)

## TOMATOES

These are a great, ripe source of vitamin C and the antioxidant lycopene, but they can cause hives and breathing difficulties in people who are allergic to aspirin because they contain salicylates, which are compounds similar to aspirin.

## 119. Potentially Harmful Herbs, Teas, and Spices

Herbs and spices, generally used in small amounts as seasonings or in teas, have a disproportionately large potential for causing allergic—and even toxic—reactions in unsuspecting individuals. All herbs and spices contain chemicals, many of which are capable of upsetting normal and essential bodily functions, especially when used in mixtures in which chemicals can potentiate each other.

**IMPORTANT** If you are taking any medication, I strongly advise consulting a nutritionally oriented doctor aware of herb–drug interactions, as even small amounts of certain herbs and spices can be dangerous in combination with particular chemicals.

## ACONITE

The fluid extract of the root of this plant is often mixed in warm water and drunk as a tea to reduce pain, fever, inflammation of the stomach, and heart palpitations. *But in the wrong proportions it can cause heart failure.*

## ALOE VERA

Though most often used as a topical ointment for healing wounds, it is frequently taken internally as a mild laxative and used in the treatment of stomach ulcers. *As an ointment it can cause hives, rashes, itching, and other allergic reactions in sensitive individuals, and it can be extremely dangerous if taken internally by pregnant women.*

## BLESSED THISTLE

Used in its proper proportions in teas to break up coughs and relieve congestion, blessed thistle is known by herbalists to live up to its name. But this is not an herb for amateurs, and unless you know how to brew it properly—don't. *High doses can cause diarrhea as well as burns of the mouth and esophagus.*

## CHAMOMILE

Frequently the tea of choice before bedtime because of its sedative, stomach-settling properties, it should be drunk in moderation. *It is a highly allergenic tea, and can cause severe allergic reactions—including fatal shock—in individuals with hay fever, or those sensitive to ragweed, asters, and related plants.*

## COMFREY

Comfrey is an herb used in teas for alleviating stomach ailments, coughs, diarrhea, arthritis, and liver and gallbladder problems. Though relatively safe, it does have a significant nutritional drawback: *Frequent ingestion can reduce your absorption of iron and vitamin $B_{12}$.*

## GREEN TEA

Green tea is rich in catechins, substances that have been shown to lower cholesterol in lab animals. Catechins have antioxidant properties that may help prevent lung and skin cancer as well as heart disease by protecting cells against damage by free radicals. And green tea also has flavor compounds that can kill *Streptococcus mutans,* bacteria involved in the formation of cavities. That said, *large doses of catechins can be toxic, and more than 2 cups a day on a regular basis are not recommended.*

## JUNIPER BERRIES

Often used as a stomach tonic, as well as a diuretic and a disinfectant of the urinary tract, juniper contains nervous system toxins. *Excessive ingestion of the berries, or beverages and tonics containing them, can cause hallucinations, among other adverse reactions.*

## LEMONS

Believe it or not, the fruit that saved innumerable sailors from scurvy, and that is used for seasoning tangy teas and thirst-quenching drinks, contains citral, a substance (also present in oranges) *that can block the beneficial activity of vitamin A.*

## LICORICE

Natural licorice, which comes from the root of a plant, contains glycyrrhizic acid. As an herb, it is often employed as a respiratory stimulant and a laxative. As a flavoring, natural licorice is often used in candy. *Consumption of large quantities (3½ ounces) daily over long periods can cause severe hypertension and cardiac arrhythmia.* (Most American licorice candy is made with synthetic flavorings and does not pose these hazards—which is just as well, since synthetic flavorings have enough of their own.)

## NUTMEG

A little sprinkled on your rice pudding won't hurt. But nutmeg, like juniper, contains nervous system toxins. *Excessive consumption can cause hallucinations, which not only won't add spice to your life, but can also endanger it.*

## PENNYROYAL

This herb, often referred to as lung mint, is frequently used as a tea for curing headaches, menstrual cramps, and pain. *It can induce abortion and should therefore never be used during pregnancy.*

## PEPPERMINT

An effective antispasmodic, peppermint tea has been used to treat nervousness, insomnia, cramps, and headaches. Though teas made from peppermint may be caffeine free, *they contain the same tannins that are in ordinary tea, which have been linked to high rates of cancer of the esophagus and stomach.*

## ROSEMARY

Taken internally, rosemary has been shown to relieve flatulence and colic, and stimulate bile release from the gallbladder. As a spice, it is a wonderful addition to salads and sauces. But a little is all you need. *Ingestion of large quantities can be toxic.*

## ST. JOHN'S WORT

Called nature's Prozac, St. John's wort has been around for centuries to heal wounds. It contains hypericin, a natural mood booster that also has germicidal and anti-inflammatory properties. It is available over the counter as dried leaves, flowers, tinctures, extract, oil, ointment, capsules, and prepared tea. *It is not recommended for long-term use without the supervision of an herbalist or other medical professional. It may cause sensitivity to light and could seriously exacerbate sunburn.*

## TARRAGON

An impressive spice that adds gourmet flavor to salads, soups, and sauces, tarragon also contains the oil estragole, *which has been shown to cause cancer in laboratory animals.*

## 120. Raw Foods That You Are Better Off Cooking

Cooking vegetables and fruits has been an anathema for nutritionists (myself included) and health-conscious individuals for years. But the times are changing. Increased concern about nutrition has fostered numerous studies that have revealed some startling new facts about the benefits of cooking food formerly held to be more nutritious raw.

### BLUEBERRIES, BLACKBERRIES, AND RED CABBAGE

Rich in vitamin $B_1$ (thiamine), which is essential for keeping the nervous system, muscles, and heart functioning normally—as well as for the proper digestion of carbohydrates—blueberries, blackberries, and red cabbage are some of the many fruits and vegetables usually eaten raw, but that can be better for you if cooked. They contain enzymes that deactivate nutrients, primarily vitamin $B_1$, when your body tries to digest them. But heat, though ordinarily an enemy of vitamin $B_1$, breaks down these enzymes and allows your body to get more of the nutrient.

### RAW PEANUTS, BEANS, AND LEGUMES

These contain enzyme inhibitors that make it difficult for your body to digest protein. Once again, heat breaks down these enzymes so you can benefit from the food's nutrients. Cooking also aids in the digestion of these foods.

## 121. Some Other Advantages of Cooking

You might want to think twice about ordering steak tartar or making sushi a regular part of your diet when I tell you that:

- Thorough cooking has been shown to be one of the most effective preventatives against food poisoning, since it can destroy salmonella bacteria.
- Cooking lowers the fat content of all meat, fish, and poultry unless, of course, you add oil in their preparation.
- Cooking helps remove many of the fat-soluble contaminants (PCBs, for instance) that collect in the fatty tissues of fish.
- Cooked meat is easier to digest because the molecules have already been partly broken down before reaching your stomach.
- Ground beef cooked over *medium* heat contains chemicals that act as anticarcinogens and help inactivate substances that are potential cancer-causing agents.

## 122. When Cooking Is Not So Hot

Though many foods might be more nutritious cooked, cooking them the wrong way can sometimes be more harmful than not eating them at all.

### COOKING CONSTERNATIONS

- Foods barbecued, flame broiled, or cooked at high temperatures are very likely to contain carcinogens.
- Cooking accelerates the oxidation of fats, producing free radical molecules that can change the metabolism and growth of body cells.
- Charcoal broiling causes the rise of smoke containing a chemical known as benzopyrene, a carcinogen, to coat the food being grilled.

**CAUTION** Charcoal broiling can speed up the metabolism of certain drugs and diminish their effectiveness. Among those found most vulnerable are antiasthmatic medications containing theophylline (Exlixophyllin, Marax, Quibron) and analgesics containing phenacetin, such as Darvon Compound, Emprazil, Fiorinal, Norgesic, and Soma Compound.

- Adding baking soda to cooking water can destroy the food's thiamine.
- Cooking salty, acidic, or alkaline food in aluminum pots can dissolve the metal so that it leaches into the food. This intensifies the cooking odors of cabbage, broccoli, and brussels sprouts and tends to turn potatoes yellowish.
- Unlined copper pots can be dangerous for cooking or storing acidic foods, or any foods cooked with wine or vinegar, as the foods can absorb this mineral, which is potentially toxic.
- Glass pots might appear hazard free, but the fact that glass lets in light can increase the loss of light-sensitive nutrients, such as vitamins $B_2$ (riboflavin), $B_{12}$ (cobalamin), $B_{13}$ (orotic acid), $B_{15}$ (pangamic acid), and C (ascorbic acid), and folic acid.
- Plastic storage containers such as margarine tubs, take-out containers, whipped-topping bowls, and other one-time-use containers should not be used in microwave ovens. These containers can warp or melt, possibly causing harmful chemicals to migrate into the food. (See section 136 for other microwave cautions.)
- Stainless steel pots are inadvisable if you're sensitive to certain metals that can leach into foods from pots when their inner surfaces have been damaged or scratched. Even minute amounts of nickel, for instance, can cause adverse reactions, as well as destroy vitamin C in foods.
- Thawing frozen vegetables before cooking depletes them of nutrients.

### 123. Cooking to Preserve Nutrients and Your Health

The best way to cook foods is fast, medium, and slow. Now, hold on: This only sounds confusing.

By fast, I mean microwaving, pressure cooking, steaming, or stir-frying, which destroy fewer nutrients while thoroughly cooking foods.

By medium, I mean the temperature at which food is cooked. High temperatures (above 400°F) tend to produce more potentially cancer-causing substances and fewer anticarcinogenic ones than medium cooking temperatures.

By slow, I mean not cooking quickly with searing heat, fast deep-frying or pan-frying, and cooking slowly over a medium flame, or roasting in a medium oven.

## SOME TIPS TO KEEP IN MIND

- Vitamin C is easily destroyed by heat and oxygen, but it doesn't have to be. If you put a vegetable, for instance, cabbage, in water that has been boiling actively for a minute or more, the water loses its vitamin-depleting oxygen and the cabbage retains all but about 2 percent of its vitamin C. (Putting cabbage in cold water, then bringing it to a boil depletes more than twelve times that amount of vitamin C.)

- Steaming vegetables, which means using a minimum amount of water, helps keep nutrients in and vegetables looking and tasting fresh instead of overcooked. (A small colander can turn any pot into a steamer.)

- Using nonstick pans allows you to get what you want out of food, nutrient-wise, without having to burden your body with unnecessary cooking fats or oils. (There are even nonstick woks available for stir-frying.)

- Cooking foods, particularly poultry, soon after purchase can halt the formation of surface bacteria that spoil food rapidly, and enable you to keep the food several days longer without having to freeze it.

- Cooking meats with vegetables that contain vitamins A, C, and E (see section 145), antioxidant vitamins, slows down the chemical deterioration of the meat and keeps it tasting fresher longer.

- Saving liquids from cooked vegetables for use in soups and gravies enables you to reclaim nutrients that were lost in the water.

## 124. Vegetarian Vulnerabilities

There are many advantages to being a vegetarian. Among them are diminished risks of coronary disease, heart attack, stroke, hypertension, and various forms of cancer, which has been attributed to vegetarians' low consumption of saturated animal fats and high consumption of fiber, whole grains, and vegetables. But there are disadvantages, too.

Vegetarian restrictions may cause anemia, impaired immunity, vitamin and mineral deficiencies, and an inability to metabolize necessary protein.

## 125. The Big $B_{12}$ Problem

Vegans, who eat no animal foods of *any* kind (no milk, cheese, eggs, dairy products) and derive their protein solely from plant sources, are very often deficient in vitamin $B_{12}$, which is essential for forming and regenerating red blood cells and preventing anemia. Unfortunately, symptoms of $B_{12}$ deficiency may not appear for five years *after* the body's stores have been depleted—which is a long time for any body to be in nutritional debt.

### SUGGESTED SOLUTIONS

- A high-potency vegetarian multivitamin–mineral tablet, vitamin $B_{12}$, 100 mcg, and a good B complex with folic acid, taken with meals twice daily.
- Including fortified soy milk, fortified nutritional yeast, and tempeh in your diet. (**Note:** Brewer's yeast, baker's yeast, and live yeast are not the same as fortified nutritional yeast and do *not* supply ample amounts of vitamin $B_{12}$.)
- Adding seaweeds, such as dulse, kelp, and spirulina (a freshwater relative), to your meals. These are prime vegetable sources of vitamin $B_{12}$, as well as other nutrients, and can be prepared in a variety of ways.

**CAUTION** Spirulina has a high phenylalanine content, and is contraindicated during pregnancy and for anyone with PKU or skin cancer.

## 126. The Amino Acid Balancing Act

Without proper balancing of amino acids through the right combination of foods, vegans may suffer from a lack of *usable* protein.

In order for effective protein synthesis to occur, there must be a balance between "essential" and "nonessential" amino acids, and the essentials in proper proportion to one another. For example, the essential amino acid lysine is needed for growth, tissue repair, and the production of antibodies, hormones, and enzymes. It is present in all protein-rich foods, including soy products, but is not in certain cereal proteins such as gliadin (from wheat) and zein (from corn). For vegetarians, this can present serious problems since wheat and corn are common dietary staples.

Lysine should be consumed in a two-to-one ratio to methionine (another essential amino acid). If not, a food that contains 100 percent of your lysine requirement but only 20 percent of your methionine will result in only 10 percent of the protein in that food being usable as protein by your body. (The remainder becomes fuel instead of body-tissue repair and building material.) Combining a lysine-rich food with another that's high in methionine solves the problem.

Vegetarians who find themselves troubled by an inability to concentrate, fatigue, bloodshot eyes, nausea, dizziness, hair loss, cold sores, and anemia are usually deficient in lysine. Methionine deficiencies, characterized by the body's inability to process urine, resulting in edema (swelling due to retention of fluids in tissues) and increased susceptibility to infection, are equally common in amino acid–imbalanced diets. (Cholesterol deposits, arteriosclerosis, and hair loss have also been linked to methionine deficiency.)

Because so many fruits and vegetables are either missing or low in amino acids, rendering those that are present relatively useless unless they are combined in a meal with foods high in those amino acids, the careful combining of complete and incomplete proteins (see section 107) is a necessity for vegetarians.

## SUGGESTED SOLUTIONS

- Vegetarian supplements. These can be obtained in liquid or powdered form and are derived from soybeans, which contain all the
  essential amino acids. Available without carbohydrates or fats,
  these supplements generally supply 26 g of protein per ounce
  (2 tablespoons), about the equivalent of a 3-ounce T-bone steak.
  Look for formulas modeled after naturally occurring proteins so
  that you can get the proper therapeutic value.

**CAUTION** It is dangerous for any supplement to be used in place of food
on a regular basis, taken in megadoses, or substituted for medication without the advice of a physician. Always keep supplements out of the reach
of children.

## 127. An Apple Today Can't Keep Doctors Away

Apples are filled with fabulous pectin fiber, along with potassium, vitamin
A, and other wholesome nutrients. Unfortunately, unless they are totally
organic, they are loaded with pesticides.

It's been ten years since the EPA finally banned the use of Alar
(daminozide) on apples, but apples are no safer now than they were then.
Alar was a potentially carcinogenic chemical pesticide used by growers to
prevent ripening apples from dropping prematurely and to increase their
storage life, that broke down with heat or digestion to form UDMH, a
potent carcinogen. *Daminozide could not be washed off or peeled away and was
absorbed inside the apple, passing on its insidious residue in all products made from
the fruit.*

For adults who consume apple products only occasionally, the risk is
considered minimal. But for infants and young children, whose bodies grow
rapidly—and who consume apple juice and other products in quantity—
the enormity of the health hazard cannot be overstated.

According to the Environmental Working Group (EWG), a series of
new analyses of government pesticide records show that every day 610,000
children (ages one through five) eat a dose of neurotoxic organophosphate

insecticides (OPs) that the government deems unsafe. And more than half of these children get that dose by eating an apple, applesauce, or apple juice!

Exposure to neurotoxic compounds such as OP insecticides (or PCBs and lead) can cause permanent, long-term damage to the brain and nervous system, especially when exposure occurs during critical periods of fetal development or early childhood. According to the EWG, the average one-year-old gets an unsafe dose of OPs approximately 2 percent of the time he or she eats just three bites of an apple sold in the United States.

How do you like them apples? I don't. To minimize your family's exposure to these chemicals, look for foods that have been certified as having exceptionally low pesticide residues, such as NutriClean certified produce, and buy as much organic food as possible.

## 128. Crudités to Consume Cautiously

As healthy and good for you as fresh vegetables are, certain wholesome crudités are not for everyone. Broccoli, brussels sprouts, cabbage, cauliflower, horseradish, kale, and turnips, among others, can interfere with thyroid function.

Consumption of large amounts of these cruciferous vegetables, which, ironically, have been shown to have impressive anticarcinogenic properties, can cause iodine-deficiency disease, goiter, thyroiditis, and hyper- or hypofunction of the thyroid gland.

If you have an underactive thyroid gland, an excessive intake of these vegetables can worsen your condition by undermining the effectiveness of such medications as Proloid, Synthroid, and similar others. In fact, if your thyroid is underactive and you're trying to lose weight, eating large amounts of these low-calorie vegetables could be the reason you can't shake those pounds. But when these vegetables are eaten in moderation, they are great sources of nutrients and are highly recommended.

## 129. Half-Truths About Whole Grains

There are few finer sources of fiber, nutrients, and complex carbohydrates than whole grains. But a lot about whole grains should be taken, literally and figuratively, with a grain of salt. (In fact, cooking grains with a pinch of salt is recommended to alkalinize their acidic properties, though a side dish containing salt and thorough chewing can perform the same function.)

## WHAT YOU SHOULD KNOW ABOUT GRAINS

- Bran is not a balanced food. (It is an indigestible complex sugar that is only part of a nutrient-balanced whole grain.)
- Oats contain the highest percentage of fat of any cultivated grain. (They also contain a natural antioxidant that retards spoilage, have been found to lower blood cholesterol levels and insulin requirements, and are a good replacement grain for individuals allergic to wheat.)
- Buckwheat groats and grits are not truly grains, and are in the same botanical family as belladonna. (They are nonetheless fine sources of vitamin E and have been found to neutralize toxic acidic wastes in the body.)
- Corn is one of the most popular but least nutritionally complete grains. (When popped, it has terrific fiber benefits; otherwise, it should be consumed with other foods to provide any significant nutrient value.)
- Rye has the highest amount of lysine, yet contains the lowest amount of whole-grain protein. (Its paucity of gluten is a plus for individuals allergic to that substance.)
- Millet is rich in minerals, has perhaps the most complete protein of all grains, and yet is generally considered grain that's strictly "for the birds." (This underappreciated grain happens to be the only one that can be boiled like rice for main dishes, used to thicken and flavor soups and stews, made into a breakfast cereal, and remain alkaline *without* the addition of salt.)
- Long-grain rice has more protein, but fewer minerals than short-grain rice. (The rices to avoid are the "instant" and "minute" varieties, which are the lowest in nutrient content.)

- All whole-grain rice is called *brown* even when it is not. (Brown rice can be cream colored, even red, but it is still the grain highest in B-complex vitamins.)
- Barley (usually available as "pearl barley") has most of its vitamins and minerals removed during milling. (This grain makes up for its nutrient deficiencies by being extremely easy to digest and adding healthy complex carbohydrate, when mixed in soups and pilafs, to the diets of sick or elderly individuals.)

**CAUTION** Excessive and exclusive consumption of whole wheat, oats, and protein-rich grains, nuts, and seeds—all of which are plentiful sources of the amino acid arginine—can be hazardous for anyone with herpes or a schizophrenic condition.

## 130. Finding Grains of Goodness

Buying whole grains without knowing what to look for in quality can rip you off nutritionally and economically.

### A GRAIN-BUYING GUIDE

1. The grains in the bin should look whole and distinct at first glance. (Consistency of milling is a sign of quality.)
2. There should be no more than a minimum amount of unhulled or greenish, immature grains.
3. Broken or damaged grains are nutrient wipeouts, and more than a minimum number in any one bin is a good indicator of the poor quality of the lot.
4. The bin should contain no extraneous matter, such as particles of dirt or stones, and the kernels for any single grain should be all about the same size or shape.
5. Test grains at home for nutritive quality by pouring a cup of them into a pot of water. Wholesome grains will sink to the

THE HAZARDS OF "HEALTH" AND HEALTHY FOODS

bottom. If more than 1 or 2 percent remain floating, you'd be wise to look for another supplier.

## 131. Getting Sour on Yogurt

In the Middle East it is known as *mast,* in Armenia *matzoon,* in Russia it is *kumyss* or *kefir,* but most of us know it as yogurt. Originally consumed here as a health food, because of its beneficial culture *Lactobacillus bulgaricus,* which is used to ferment or curdle the milk with which it is made, yogurt has now become almost as popular as ice cream—and in some cases just about as nutritious.

Yes, there are lots of good things to say about yogurt, but that doesn't mean all of them are true. In fact, there are a lot of "yes-buts" about yogurt that most people don't know.

**Yes ...**

Yogurt is a good food for dieters.

**But ...**

It is *not* nonfattening. Plain whole-milk yogurt has virtually the same number of calories as the milk used to make it. (One cup of whole milk has 150 calories; a cup of plain whole-milk yogurt has approximately 140 calories— and some commercial brands have even more.)

Yogurt helps digestion and replaces friendly bacteria that are often destroyed during antibiotic therapies.

All brands of yogurt do not contain these beneficial bacterial cultures because many manufacturers pasteurize the yogurt *after* culturing, destroying the bacteria to extend the shelf life of their product.

| **Yes . . .** | **But . . .** |
|---|---|
| Yogurt is nutritious. | It is not a complete meal any more than a glass of milk is. In fact, yogurt is slightly lower in vitamins A and C, folic acid, and magnesium than fortified milk. Unless yogurt is eaten with fresh vegetables or fruit, it's little more than a wholesome snack. |
| Yogurt is pure and natural. | Only if it is homemade, or among a select few plain (unflavored) commercially marketed brands. Most contain stabilizers and other additives. Fruit-filled or "naturally flavored" yogurts contain added sweeteners (which are sometimes listed separately or covered under the heading "selected preserves" on labels), and often potassium sorbate, modified food starch, and artificial colors and flavors as well. |
| Frozen yogurt has much less fat than ice cream. | It has about the same number of calories because of its added sweeteners. |

## 132. What They Forgot to Tell You at the Health Food Store

A little bit of knowledge can be a dangerous thing when it comes to foods and supplements consumed primarily for health benefits. Being unaware of how even the most beneficial products from nature's pantry can backfire for you is not just asking for trouble—it is ensuring it.

## ABOUT GINSENG

Ginseng is an authentic, natural, mental and physical stimulant that helps assimilate vitamins and minerals. Often called manroot because of its resemblance to the human body, it has been used around the world for centuries as a natural "upper" and an aphrodisiac. (Because of its normalizing effect on the body's metabolism, it reduces stress, which can contribute significantly to sexual performance and pleasure.) Unfortunately, many ginseng users never benefit from it. This is because they are rarely informed that high doses of vitamin C—and foods rich in vitamin C—can inhibit its effectiveness. Taking ginseng three hours before or after a vitamin C supplement, or C-rich foods, should correct this. (Also, taking a time-release vitamin C supplement makes counteractions less likely.)

## ABOUT GARLIC

Garlic has been found to contain substances that reduce high blood pressure, help combat diabetes by cleaning the blood of excess glucose (which is not to suggest it be used to replace medically prescribed methods), increase immunity to bronchial infections, aid in fighting certain types of cancer, lower blood cholesterol levels, and help in the prevention of heart disease. But it is the *oils* of these bulbs that contain the therapeutic properties. If the "odorless" pills you have been buying contain only garlic powder, you're getting a nutritional brush-off. Look for perles containing extracts of fresh garlic. They are just as odorless because they dissolve in the lower intestine, not in the stomach. But if you're concerned about your breath, taking a few natural chlorophyll tablets (which happen to have antibacterial properties that go beyond bad breath) should solve the problem.

## ABOUT YEAST

Yeast is an excellent source of protein, a superior source of the natural B-complex vitamins (with the exception of $B_{12}$, which is bred only into fortified nutritional yeast), organic iron, trace minerals, and amino acids. But like other protein foods, yeast is high in phosphorus, which means that to reap its benefits without jeopardizing your health you should be adding extra calcium to your diet. Too much phosphorus, in case you have forgotten, can take calcium *out* of the body. And if you want your nutritional pluses from yeast to *really* rise, take a balanced B-complex supplement along with it. Together they work like a powerhouse.

## ABOUT CAROB

Carob is a terrific alternative to chocolate because it is caffeine free and is much lower in fat. (Carob powder has less than 0.5 g fat as opposed to cocoa powder's 3 to 5.5 g.) But by the time the manufacturers turn carob powder into carob coating for candy, they have added enough oil so that these so-called health treats have as much if not more fat per ounce than almost any commercial chocolate bar.

## ABOUT SAFFLOWER OIL

Safflower oil has the highest percentage of unsaturated fats and is highest in linoleic acid (found to aid in combating cholesterol deposits and heart disease, protecting against the harmful effects of x-rays, and promoting healthy skin and hair). But most buyers aren't told that it spoils easily, requires refrigeration in warm climates, and should not be used for deep-frying because its flavor is unstable under high temperatures.

## ABOUT SOYBEAN OIL

Soybean oil is a strong seller—with a strong flavor—with vegetarians. The kind sold in health food stores is unrefined and highly susceptible to oxidation. Though often used in salad dressings, foods fried in it develop off-flavors quickly. (If you are going to fry food, I would recommend sesame oil. It's mild in flavor, 87 percent unsaturated, not prone to quick oxidation, and tastes good, too.)

## ABOUT POLYUNSATURATED OILS

All of them aren't the same, and though all contain high amounts of linoleic acid (necessary for producing the lecithin that lowers blood cholesterol levels), many are refined to the point that they are virtually depleted of vitamin E and other nutrients. Since the amount of vitamin E that you need is directly proportional to the amount of polyunsaturates you consume, a polyunsaturated oil with its vitamin E removed can, in effect, create a ready-made vitamin E deficiency.

## 133. Any Questions About Chapter 10?

*My husband and I are vegetarians, and occasionally make meatless burgers from mixes that I get at the health food store. They don't seem to bother him, but I break out in hives, or get flushed and itchy, mostly on nights that we eat them. Do natural meat analogs contain substances that can cause allergic reactions?*

They do indeed, especially if you are allergic to any grains, such as wheat, oats, barley, millet, or legumes (soybeans, peas, lentils), or nuts, which are often used in varying combinations in meat analogs. Check ingredients carefully, because many also add egg to their formulas along with different dehydrated vegetables. In fact, some imply they are totally natural (and may even be labeled as such) and are sold in health food stores even though they contain carrageenan, MSG, artificial flavors, and other additives—any of which might be causing your after-dinner discomforts.

*Is there any way to tell if the yogurt I'm eating really has the live cultures I want for replacing the good bacteria in my system?*

Mix a few tablespoons of your plain yogurt with a cup of warmed (not boiled) milk. Leave the mixture overnight in a warm place (over the pilot light on the range will do). If your yogurt passes the test and has live cultures (probiotics), the milk will have thickened somewhat by morning. If your yogurt fails, the milk will just be . . . well, milk.

Your best bet is to buy yogurt that contains inulin. Inulin is a prebiotic, meaning it is scientifically proven to increase the activity of the beneficial bacteria as well as help prevent the growth of harmful bacteria in the digestive tract. (A natural dietary fiber, it is present in common fruits and vegetables such as artichokes, asparagus, onions, raisins, and bananas.) Inulin is a good source of soluble dietary fiber, fine for diabetics because it doesn't increase the glucose or insulin level in the blood, boosts the absorption of calcium, and helps protect against bacteria that cause many food-borne illnesses, such as *E. coli*, salmonella, staphylococcus, and listeria.

**I've heard that frozen vegetables have more vitamins than fresh ones. Could this possibly be true?**

In many cases it is. Vegetables begin to lose vitamins, particularly vitamin C, as soon as they're picked. By freezing or even canning them immediately, more vitamins are retained than if they are exposed to lengthy storage and shipping time (yes, in spite of losses incurred by processing). Frozen vegetables, though, retain more vitamins than those that are canned, because vitamins, especially water-soluble ones, are more nutritionally stable in cold than in heat.

**I use walnuts quite often in salads and breads, so to save time I buy them already shelled. Are they any less nutritious this way?**

They are not only less nutritious, they are more potentially hazardous to your health. Because of their high oil content, the removal of their shells leaves them vulnerable to rancidity. And depending on how they are processed, you are left vulnerable to the fumigants that are used in their preparation.

Ethylene gas, the fumes of which are irritating to membranes and the ingestion of which can cause liver and kidney damage, is generally used to loosen the walnuts from their shells. After shelling, the nuts are protected from spoilage (though you're not) by methylbromide, which is a potential central nervous system depressant, and then blanched by a dip in hot dye or glycerine and sodium carbonate, which in excessive amounts has been shown to increase acidity and cause serious kidney damage in dogs. Since color is considered important to sales, walnuts are also often bleached with chloride of lime and sodium carbonate.

If you're buying shelled nuts, I would suggest you steer clear of those that have been overly processed. Natural food stores are your best bet for purchasing these. Look for solid kernels. If they feel soft or rubbery, the nuts are probably old and possibly rancid. Avoid any kernels with insides that are beginning to turn gray. This is an indication that oils are coming out and rancidity has begun.

### *What's the difference between parboiled, polished, and converted white rice?*

Polished white rice, the sort you get in most Chinese restaurants, is rice that has been depleted of a large portion of its nutrients, particularly B vitamins, through a process that is used to make its protein more digestible. (This is a dubious trade-off for Westerners, whose diets are generally oversupplied with protein.)

Parboiled and converted white rice, on the other hand, is processed so that nutrients in the bran (outer layer) are essentially pushed into the endosperm, thereby retaining many more of the grain's natural vitamins and minerals.

### *What precisely is the big difference between soluble and insoluble fiber?*

To be as precise as possible, soluble fiber interferes with the absorption of fats and slows down the absorption of carbohydrates into the body. (Examples: oat bran, legumes, citrus fruits.) Insoluble fiber is a tougher variety. It doesn't break down in water, but it does absorb it, causing waste to move through and out at a quicker pace. (Examples: wheat bran, whole grains, beans.)

The important point to remember is that the more refined a food is, the less fiber it has. In other words, applesauce would have half as much fiber as a raw apple, and white bread has about eight times less than whole wheat.

## FOOD FOR THOUGHT

- Brown rice, already rich in nutrients, can be boosted in nutritional value by soaking it. Japanese researchers found that soaking rice for a day triggers germination, which activates enzymes beneficial to humans. The soaked rice had three times the amount of lysine (see section 126) and ten times more gamma-aminobutyric acid (GABA, a neurotransmitter that helps regulate nerve cells). White rice does not germinate after any amount of soaking.

- Although natural products are *generally* lower in sodium and sugar, a single prepared food item may still have more than most people should consume in a day. Consumer demand for low-fat foods has caused manufacturers to make up for the lost taste of fat by adding extra ingredients such as spices, sugar, or salt.

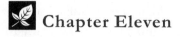 Chapter Eleven

# Cautions à la Carte

### 134. Food Poisoning Is Alive and Well

Foods deteriorate because of microbiological, physical, chemical, or enzyme-induced decay. Food processing, for better or worse, can eliminate or reduce natural and added toxins, destroy harmful parasites, and maintain nutrient quality and flavor. Nonetheless, food poisoning is still alive and well and killing people every year—mostly because of human error.

#### COMMON TYPES OF FOOD POISONING

**Botulism**   This type of food poisoning is caused by eating food that contains poison or toxin produced by bacteria growing *in the food*. Though rare (about ten to fifteen cases annually in the United States) botulism can be, and frequently is, deadly. Most cases are the result of improperly home-canned foods, although a few have been traced to commercially processed foods.

*Symptoms:* Mild stomach upset and general malaise usually appear some eighteen to forty-eight hours after eating the poisoned food. These are followed quickly by dizziness and headache, with blurred or double vision; general muscular weakness; difficulty in swallowing and speaking; respiratory failure; and coma. Death is caused by respiratory paralysis. (The odds of survival depend on the amount of poison ingested in relation to the person's body weight and how quickly emergency treatment is provided.)

If botulism is suspected, the victim should be given absolutely nothing by mouth and rushed to the hospital. Antitoxin is not always available at hospitals, but can be obtained by having your doctor phone the twenty-four-hour botulism hotline at the Centers for Disease Control and Prevention in Atlanta for information on the nearest supply. The line is for use *only by physicians* who have diagnosed the case.

*Prevention tips:*

- Never eat or even taste food from a swollen can or jar.
- If the contents of any can or jar are foamy, moldy, or have a bad color, dispose of them *immediately*. (Be sure there's no chance they will even be *tasted* by pets.)
- Never taste home-canned vegetables before cooking them. (Letting them boil for a few minutes will destroy any botulism bacteria.)
- If you are unsure of how to go about home canning, contact your local Agricultural Extension Service for reliable information—or else can the idea completely.

## STAPHYLOCOCCAL FOOD POISONING

More common, but less dangerous than botulism, this type is also caused by eating food containing poison or toxin produced by bacteria growing *in the food.* (**Note:** For infants, the elderly, and anyone suffering from other illnesses, this type of food poisoning can be *fatal.*) The staphylococcus bacteria are harmful only when allowed to contaminate and multiply in food that has been improperly stored, cooked, or handled.

*Symptoms:* Nausea, general malaise, vomiting, and/or diarrhea usually appear anywhere from one to six hours after eating a food contaminated with staphylococcus. Vomiting need not be induced, but should not be inhibited, mainly because vomiting and diarrhea can rid your body of the toxin within a day or two. When initial symptoms subside, you can drink warm mild fluids (broth, tea, and so on) and then stay on a bland diet for a few days. Special medications are not generally recommended, but you should check with your physician to be sure.

*Prevention tips:*

- Don't eat raw meat.
- Keep raw foods refrigerated. (If poultry or meat is contaminated with staphylococcus, the bacteria will multiply rapidly at room temperature—and the staphylococcus toxin is *not* destroyed by heating.)
- Thaw meat and poultry in the refrigerator, microwave, or in plastic wrap under cold water, quickly.

## SALMONELLOSIS

This type of food poisoning is an infection caused by eating food containing organisms that multiply *in the body*. It is often caused by undercooked poultry, insufficiently reheated leftovers, raw or rare meat, contaminated eggs or dairy products, or putting warm stuffing into a raw turkey and allowing it to remain uncooked (even though refrigerated) overnight. (The cold cannot penetrate the center of the turkey fast enough to kill rapidly multiplying salmonella.) Frequently misdiagnosed as an intestinal virus, the diarrheal infection caused by this bacteria may leave a legacy of serious chronic ailments, such as arthritis, kidney damage, heart problems, and intestinal damage that interferes with the ability to absorb nutrients, leaving victims with impaired immunity to numerous other illnesses.

*Symptoms:* Abdominal cramps, watery diarrhea, chills, and possibly fever can appear anywhere from six hours to a couple of days after eating the contaminated food because it takes time for the bacteria to grow in your intestinal tract. A physician should be called, since the infection could be dangerous and lead to complications. Antibiotics may or may not be required, depending on your doctor's assessment of the condition. (Frighteningly, new research indicates that many strains of salmonella bacteria have become antibiotic resistant, making the infection more dangerous today than in the past.) Diagnosis is generally confirmed by a stool sample.

*Prevention tips:*

- Scrub all surfaces on which you cut raw poultry before putting any other food there.
- Wash your hands and utensils after cutting raw poultry or meat before handling other food.
- Cook all poultry thoroughly. (The internal temperature of ground chicken and turkey—as well as that of stuffing—must reach 165°F to kill salmonella bacteria.) Boneless roasts and breast meat should be cooked to 170°F; whole birds, thighs, and drumsticks to 180°F.
- Keep foods either hot (above 165°F) or cold (below 40°F), and don't let them stand at in-between temperatures, particularly warm ones, for more than two hours.
- Don't let hot foods cool on the counter. Gradual cooling allows prime time for salmonella growth. Food should be cooled to 40°F within four hours. (If you've made a large pot of stew or chili that won't cool fast enough, divide it into smaller containers.)
- Never leave meat or poultry to defrost on the counter.
- Don't use eggs that have cracks in them.

**SEAFOOD POISONING**

There are two types of seafood poisoning: mytilotoxism, which comes from eating mollusks such as mussels, clams, and oysters that have fed on certain toxic microorganisms; and ciguatera poisoning, which can be caused by eating any contaminated seafood. Both types are serious and potentially fatal.

*Symptoms:* For mytilotoxism, symptoms appear very quickly, usually within half an hour. Nausea and vomiting are followed by paralysis that begins in the outer extremities and spreads to the rest of the body. Emergency treatment is required. If vomiting hasn't occurred, it should be induced, and the victim taken to the hospital. If you or others have eaten shellfish along with the victim, induce vomiting and proceed immediately to the hospital—even if no symptoms are apparent.

Symptoms of ciguatera poisoning usually appear in three to five hours. They include nausea, fatigue, giddiness, and increased salivation and sweating. Headache, dizziness, and difficulty in breathing follow. Respiratory failure can occur if the victim is not given emergency treatment. CPR or other respiratory resuscitation may be required en route to the hospital.

*Prevention tips:*

- Don't eat your own catch if you don't know what your own catch has been eating. (Commercial fisheries have much better surveillance and knowledge of what they bring in from the sea. Buy only from reputable suppliers, however, who know where their fish are coming from.)
- Don't eat raw shellfish, especially from the Gulf Coast.
- Avoid grouper, amberjack, and red snapper in tropical areas. (See section 111 for other fish cautions.)

**COMMENTS AND CAUTIONS** Ciguatera toxin is found in fish harvested from reef areas. Scombroid poisoning comes from histamine that can form on the flesh of fresh tuna, mahi mahi, and some other fish that aren't kept cold enough before they reach the market. *Neither is destroyed by heat.*

## 135. Protecting Yourself at Home and in Restaurants

Eliminating all the bacteria that cause food poisoning is impossible, but stopping their growth, killing them at the proper time, and preventing them from doing their dirty work are not.

### PRECAUTIONS FOR ALL OCCASIONS

- Never taste meat, poultry, or fish while it is cooking. (All it takes is a spoonful of uncooked bouillabaisse to let an unwanted parasite slip through your lips or put a germ of your own in the pot.)

- Avoid using the same spoon more than once for tasting food while preparing, cooking, or serving it.
- Never eat or serve food directly from a jar or can; saliva may contaminate the remaining food. (This can be particularly hazardous for infants.)
- Always keep uncooked and cooked foods containing eggs in the refrigerator.
- In foods that will *not* be cooked, use only *pasteurized* eggs, never raw eggs. (Pasteurized eggs can be found in some supermarkets, or by calling 1-800-447-3447.)
- Don't hold food for more than two to three hours in an automatic oven before cooking.
- Cutting boards, meat grinders, blenders, and can openers should be washed thoroughly after each use. (Chlorine laundry bleach in the proportion recommended on the package is effective at destroying bacteria.)
- Have two cutting boards. Delegate one (not made of wood) for raw meats, fish, and poultry—and wash it immediately after use in hot soapy water.
- Never partially cook meat or poultry one day and complete cooking the next.
- Always wash your hands with hot soapy water before cooking and eating. (The worst organisms for food-borne illnesses are fecally transmitted.) Wash under rings and fingernails. Dry with a disposable towel.
- Keep raw meats, fish, and poultry in their original packages and place them on plates on the bottom shelf in the refrigerator to prevent juices from dripping on other foods.
- Never handle cooked food with utensils or plates that held raw food unless they've been thoroughly washed.
- Be wary of eating food that has been prepared by someone smoking. (Smoking hazards aside, saliva might have gotten on the person's fingers, from the cigarette between her lips, and it can transmit unwanted bacteria to you.)

- Avoid restaurants where soups are served warm instead of hot, and salads tepid instead of chilled. (The longer food sits in temperatures conducive to bacterial growth, the more likely the presence of harmful bacteria.)
- If you buy prewashed, or "triple-washed" salad greens, wash them again. (You don't know what was in the water with which they were originally washed.)
- Even wash produce that you intend to peel, such as bananas, oranges, melons, and avocados, particularly if you don't intend to eat them right away. (The skin could be contaminated and when you cut the fruit, food-poisoning organisms could spread to the flesh.)
- Disinfect sponges—which can harbor all sorts of organisms—in chlorine bleach or by microwaving them on high for one minute, and replace them when worn.
- Use a refrigerator thermometer to be sure that your refrigerator is always below 40°F and your freezer is at or below 0°F.
- Read and follow the "safe handling instructions" now required by the USDA on all packaged poultry and meat.

## 136. Microwave Cooking Safety

Microwave ovens are great for retaining nutrients, especially in vegetables, because food requires minimum cooking time and minimum water. But special care must be taken when cooking or reheating meat, poultry, fish, and eggs. Microwaves can cook unevenly and leave "cold spots," where harmful bacteria can survive.

### SAFE NUKING TIPS

- Arrange food items evenly in a covered dish (add liquid if needed). Cover with a lid or plastic wrap; loosen or vent the wrap to let steam escape. The moist heat that's created will help destroy harmful bacteria and ensure uniform cooking.

- Stir or rotate food midway through microwaving to eliminate cold spots.
- Cook large cuts of meat on medium (50 percent) power to allow heat to reach the center without overcooking the outer areas.
- If partially cooking food in the microwave to finish cooking on a grill or in a conventional oven, transfer microwaved food to the other heat source immediately. Never partially cook food and store it for later use.
- Avoid cooking whole, stuffed poultry in a microwave oven. The stuffing might not reach the temperature needed to destroy harmful bacteria.
- Before checking the internal temperature with a food thermometer, always allow standing time, which completes the cooking.
- Before defrosting, remove food from packaging.
- Do not use foam trays or plastic wraps because they are not heat stable—and melting may cause harmful chemicals to leach into the food.
- Cook defrosted meat, poultry, egg dishes, and fish immediately after defrosting in the microwave because some areas of the frozen food may begin to cook during the defrosting time.
- When reheating foods, cover with a lid or microwave plastic wrap. Allow standing time and then check to see that food has reached 165°F.
- Heat all ready-to-eat foods (hot dogs, luncheon meats, and leftovers) until steaming hot.
- Use only cookware specially manufactured for microwave use.
- Do not let plastic wrap touch foods during microwaving.
- Never use plastic storage bags, brown paper or plastic grocery bags, newspapers, or aluminum foil in a microwave oven.

## 137. Is That Still Okay to Eat?

How many times have you opened your refrigerator, freezer, or pantry and wondered whether something was still okay to eat, and wound up convincing yourself that it was? How many times have you told yourself, "When in doubt, throw it out" and have?

If you have done more of the eating than the throwing out, you're playing a risky nutritional game. Foods don't have to be toxic to sabotage your body. They can quite efficiently undermine you physically and emotionally simply by depriving you of nutrients, or by sneakily plying you with relatively harmless bacteria that slowly but surely can weaken your immune system, leaving you vulnerable to innumerable, avoidable ailments.

Keeping yourself out of nutritional danger is knowing what and when foods could be harmful—and not eating them.

## 138. Learn the Dating Game

Most processed foods are still dated in a code that only the manufacturer can decipher. Some perishable foods, however, are required by law to have what is known as an "open date" that consumers can understand. Unfortunately, there are four kinds of open dates ("blind dates" would be a more appropriate description), and it's a rare consumer who understands any of them. But learning how can make a big difference to your health.

### TRANSLATIONS FOR CONSUMERS

- Dairy products, cold cuts, fresh fruit juices, and bakery goods usually have a "sell by" date, indicating that the product should not be sold after that date (though bakery goods often are, at reduced prices).

*Translation:* Unless the product can be frozen, you shouldn't keep it for more than two to three days.

- Canned and frozen foods have a "packed on" date, which isn't too helpful unless you know how long the food will remain fresh, which most of us don't.

*Translation:* Use the frozen foods within three to four months of the date, canned foods within a year. There is no health danger in keeping them longer, but there is no nutritional point to it, either.

- Products marked "best if used by" mean that the manufacturer backs their quality and freshness up to that date.

*Translation:* It is not dangerous to use the product after the date—unless, of course, it turns moldy (see section 139)—but don't count on getting the same nutrition from it.

- Any foods that have an "expiration (EXP)" date should be taken seriously. If the manufacturer doesn't want you to eat it, that's a good enough reason not to do so.

*Translation:* If you've passed the date, dump the product.

## 139. Mind Those Molds

The refrigerator is a great spawning ground for molds because they can tolerate low temperatures. But these greenish-grayish intruders are not budding penicillin sources; they are powerful troublemakers that can accelerate food spoilage and produce poisons.

### MUST-KNOWS ABOUT MOLD

- Never sniff moldy food. (Molds can cause allergic reactions and produce respiratory problems.)
- Foods heavily covered with mold should be carefully wrapped in a paper towel (you don't want any seditious spores let loose in your refrigerator) and discarded immediately. The area where the moldy food was should be cleaned thoroughly and all nearby foods carefully examined.
- A small moldy spot on cheese, hard salami, or smoked turkey can be cut off and the food saved, provided you cut off *at least an inch around and below the mold spot,* and rewrap the food in fresh paper. (Moldy bacon, hot dogs, sliced luncheon meats, meat pies, canned hams, and baked chicken should be thrown out.)
- Spots of surface mold on firm vegetables, such as carrots and cabbage, can be cut away and the vegetables will still be safe to eat

raw or cooked. Soft vegetables (tomatoes, cucumbers, lettuce, and so on) should be discarded if they show signs of mold growth.

- Discard any moldy soft cheese, cottage cheese, cream, sour cream, yogurt, and individual cheese slices.
- Moldy bread as well as other baked goods should be discarded. (If one slice of bread has begun to green, you can be sure the mold is working its way through the loaf.)
- Dried nuts, beans, rice, whole grains, flour, corn, and peanut butter should be tossed out if there are signs of mold, as they can be extremely hazardous to your health.

## 140. Possible Plastic Problems

Ever since a scientist at Tufts University found that breast cancer cells proliferated in new plastic test tubes, and that the reaction was caused by a compound in polyvinylchloride (PVC) and polystyrene plastics that migrated from the plastic to the cells, plastic containers and food wraps have become a health concern. And although the FDA has deemed them safe, the public verdict is still out on their potential for negatively impacting our bodies.

"Plasticizers," chemicals added to plastic to make it softer, are suspected of being hormone disrupters. The prime suspect chemical, di (2-ethylhexyl) phthalate (DEHP), a compound found in deli-style cling wrap and household wraps such as Reynolds and Saran Wrap, was found to migrate into cheese during a Consumers Union test. (In animal studies, even small amounts of hormone disrupters have been found to cause genetic abnormalities or cancer.) But DEHP, formerly classified as "possibly carcinogenic for humans" by the International Agency for Research on Cancer (IARC) based on the animal studies, was reclassified in February 2000 by that same agency as "not classifiable as to carcinogenicity to humans," conceding that while it does cause tumors in rodents, its action is not relevant to humans.

My feeling is that if it's not okay for Mickey Mouse, it's not okay for me. Until the final word is in, the best thing to do is to play it safe with plastics. Phthalates like DEHP are fat soluble and easily absorbed from packaging materials by high-fat foods such as cheese, butter, and lunch meats.

## PLASTIC PRECAUTIONS

- Rewrap deli cheese and meats in aluminum foil or wax paper. If you prefer plastic wrap, use a polyethylene wrap, such as America's Choice, Glad Crystal, Foodtown, Duane Reede, or White Rose. (Polyethylene lacks plasticizers.)
- Don't store food for extended periods in Styrofoam containers. The styrene molecules migrate into the food. (Foods will actually develop a plastic taste.)
- Be aware that extreme heat (microwaving) and cold (refrigeration) increase migration of styrene into food—with acidic and fatty foods absorbing more of it than other foods.
- Throw out old plastic containers that show signs of wear.
- Avoid even microwave-safe plastic containers and use glass or glass ceramic (for example, Corningware) for microwaving.
- If you buy foods wrapped in plastic, scrape the surface layer of the food before eating or cooking to remove any possible contamination.

**COMMENTS AND CAUTIONS** Phthalates can be easily absorbed, ingested, and inhaled. They are found not only in plastic wraps, but also in toys, teethers, and baby bottles. The Environmental Health Network of California has petitioned the FDA to require labeling on perfumes (such as Calvin Klein's "Eternity") that contain phthalates. Additionally, recent research has found that phthalates leaching out of old Barbie dolls may disrupt hormone development and be a contributing factor to early puberty among females who've spent hours playing with Barbie dolls. And when polyvinyl chloride (PVC) plastic toys, which have toxic chemical additives, are chewed or sucked, children are even more at risk for future health problems. Because it's better to be safe than sick, my advice is to avoid plastic products that contain phthalates as much as possible.

## 141. How Long Will It Keep?

- Raisins in an airtight container, in a cool place, will keep in prime condition for more than six months.
- Grapes will stay fresh in the refrigerator for three to five days.
- Herbs and spices have volatile oils that oxidize easily. If stored in small jars, tightly covered, and kept away from heat, humidity, and light, they'll keep nicely for at least a year.
- Whole-wheat flour will usually go rancid within one to two months unless stored in the refrigerator or frozen.
- A peanut butter sandwich will keep for two days without refrigeration.
- Cooked wild rice will keep for only a week in the refrigerator, but will last several months if frozen.
- Beer in cans will begin to deteriorate in three months; in bottles, in five months.
- Nuts will keep for a year or longer if frozen in tightly closed containers.
- Cooked beans, tightly covered, will keep for up to five days in the refrigerator.
- Eggplant will keep fresh for about a week.
- Green onions and chives should be refrigerated and used within a few days after purchase.
- Soft unripened cheeses, such as cottage, cream, or Neufchâtel, should be refrigerated and used within a few days after purchase or of the "sell by" date.
- Ripened and cured cheese will keep in the refrigerator for several weeks if protected from mold contamination.
- Though many cheeses are damaged by freezing, certain varieties can be frozen for six months if they are cut into small pieces (not over an inch thick) or grated, and wrapped in moisture-proof

freezer paper or stored in airtight containers. (Cheeses that are among those most suitable for freezing in small pieces are brick, Camembert, cheddar, Edam, Gouda, mozzarella, Muenster, Port du Salut, provolone, and Swiss.)

- Fresh-chilled or packaged poultry should be used within one to two days of purchase.
- Fresh prepackaged meat should be stored, unopened, in the refrigerator in the original wrapping no longer than two days. (Larger cuts, such as roasts, may stay three to four days.) Without rewrapping, meat will stay fresh in the freezer for one to two weeks. (For longer storage, the package must be overwrapped with special freezer paper or foil.)
- Frozen meat should be stored at 0°F or lower immediately after purchase to prevent loss of quality and bacterial growth.
- Fresh meat should be used within two to four days of purchase for optimum quality.
- Ground meats should be used within one to two days.
- Fresh beef should be kept frozen no longer than a year.
- Fresh veal and lamb should be kept frozen no longer than nine months.
- Fresh pork should be kept frozen no longer than six months.
- Ground beef, veal, and lamb should be kept frozen no longer than four months.
- Ground pork should be kept frozen no longer than three months.
- Fresh pork sausage should be used within one week or kept frozen no longer than sixty days. (Smoked sausage should be used within three to seven days.)
- Bacon and frankfurters will keep five to seven days in the refrigerator; one month in the freezer.
- A whole smoked ham will keep one week in the refrigerator; two months in the freezer.
- Ham slices will keep three to four days in the refrigerator; two months in the freezer.

- Corned beef will keep one week in the refrigerator; two weeks in the freezer.
- Leftover cooked meat will keep four to five days in the refrigerator; two to three months in the freezer.

## 142. Portions of Cautions

No matter how nutritious a food is and how important individual nutrients are, there will always be times, situations, and metabolic conditions where cautions and special adjustments are advised. I suggest that you read the following list carefully for your own well-being. It can help you reap benefits and sidestep risks that may often be just opposite sides of the same nutritional coin.

- Whole-wheat flour contains difficult-to-digest carbohydrates that are attacked by bacteria in the large intestine, frequently causing gas and diarrhea.
- Many salt substitutes contain potassium chloride, which can be hazardous in large amounts and should not be used without first consulting your physician or a nutritionally oriented doctor.
- Overconsumption of vitamin $B_1$ (thiamine) can affect thyroid and insulin production, and might cause loss of other B vitamins. (See section 145 for natural sources of thiamine.)
- An insufficiency of vitamin A in your diet can lead to loss of vitamin C and a weakened immune system.
- Don't eat raw eggplant; it could contain toxic solanine. (Cooking destroys solanine.)
- Ingestion of large amounts of vitamin $B_2$ (riboflavin) without sufficient amounts of vitamins A, C, and E and selenium in your diet may cause sensitivity to sunlight.
- Don't eat raw egg whites. They deactivate the body's biotin.
- Large doses of vitamin C wash out $B_{12}$ and folic acid, so be careful about taking C supplements—particularly if you are a

vegetarian—without the compensation of sufficient $B_{12}$ and folic acid to meet your minimum requirements.

- If you have a medical history of convulsive disorders or hormone-related cancer, high intakes of folic acid for extended periods of time are not recommended.
- Excessive consumption of foods rich in PABA (para-aminobenzoic acid) can have a negative effect on the liver, kidneys, and heart in certain individuals.
- Anyone with sickle-cell anemia, hemochromatosis, or thalassemia should not take iron supplements, eat large amounts of iron-rich foods, or eat food cooked in cast-iron pots.
- Large amounts of caffeine from coffee, colas, or chocolate can inhibit iron absorption and also create an inositol shortage in the body.
- Anyone with kidney malfunction should not eat large quantities of magnesium-rich foods. Over 3,000 mg daily can be dangerous. (Keep in mind that just 2 cups of roasted almonds supply more than 700 mg.)
- Milk is not a good source of iron, which is necessary for the metabolization of B vitamins.
- It is possible that large amounts of vitamin C might reverse the anticoagulant activity of the blood thinner warfarin, commonly prescribed as the drug Coumadin.
- Anyone taking thyroid medication should be aware that kelp also affects that gland. If you have been using both, a consultation with your doctor is advisable. You might need *less* prescription medicine than you think.
- If you take cortisone or aldosterone drugs (for example, Aldactone, Prednisone) you *lose* potassium and retain sodium. Check with your doctor for proper diet restructuring and supplements.
- If you're trying to increase the zinc in your diet, be sure you are getting enough vitamin A for it to be effective.
- Foods high in folic acid and PABA inhibit the effectiveness of sulfonamides such as Gantrisin.

- Large amounts of raw cabbage can cause an iodine deficiency and throw off thyroid production in individuals with existing low-iodine intakes.
- Milk that contains synthetic vitamin D can deplete the body of magnesium.
- The artificial sweetener aspartame (NutraSweet) contains phenyl-alanine, which may raise blood pressure, and should *not* be used by anyone taking MAO inhibitors.
- If you eat a lot of protein, be sure your diet includes a substantial amount of B-complex vitamins. (Surprisingly, even $B_{12}$, which is ample in high-protein foods, is also necessary because it works synergistically with the other B vitamins.)
- If you drink alcohol regularly, be sure that you're getting substantial amounts of vitamin $B_{12}$ in your diet.
- If you eat out a lot, you need to add more calcium to your diet.
- If you have an ulcer, keep away from papaya and raw pineapple, and don't use papain as a food tenderizer.
- Excessive zinc intake can result in iron and copper losses.
- Anyone suffering from Wilson's disease is susceptible to copper toxicity.
- Don't boil fluoridated water more than ten minutes. (Boiling drives off chlorine and other contaminants, but it concentrates the fluorides to an unhealthy degree.)
- Eating large mouthfuls of food can be particularly hazardous if you're taking tranquilizers such as Compazine and Thorazine, since these drugs tend to reduce the ability to cough.
- Don't eat foods that are high in purines if you are prone to gout attacks. (Purines are found mainly in fatty meats and poultry, scallops, anchovies, clams, organ meats, and vegetables such as spinach, lentils, mushrooms, peas, and asparagus, as well as in condiments, rich pastries, fried foods, and alcohol.)
- Some antihypertension medications can cause a buildup of potassium, while others (particularly thiazide diuretics) deplete it. Be sure you know which your drug is doing and consult

your doctor about adjusting your diet and supplements accordingly.

- The gluten in wheat, rye, and barley may aggravate arthritic conditions in certain individuals, and is contraindicated for anyone with celiac disease.
- Calcium can interfere with the effectiveness of tetracycline.
- Too much manganese can reduce the utilization of your body's iron.
- If you go off the Pill in order to become pregnant, do *not* eat large amounts of vitamin A–rich foods (see section 145) or take vitamin A supplements, but *do* increase the folic acid in your diet. (Too much vitamin A and too little folic acid have, under these circumstances, been associated with birth defects.)
- Iodine can worsen a dermatological condition, so avoid highly salted foods (see section 110) and any that use iodized salt.
- Heavy milk drinkers and meat eaters need to increase the manganese in their diets.
- High-protein, low-carbohydrate diets can diminish your production of two essential hormones: thyroid and norepinephrine.
- Suddenly stopping a high-protein, low-carbohydrate diet can cause a rapid drop in potassium and magnesium, and result in heart rhythm irregularity.
- Chocolate can cause anal itching.
- Avoid mixed baby food dinners that might contain modified food starch. Many young infants cannot digest starches. Undigested starches can cause diarrhea, which can keep an infant from absorbing necessary nutrients.
- Tomatoes should not be left to ripen in the sun. They'll lose most of their vitamin C and other nutrients.
- Bulgur wheat is not a whole-wheat product unless the granules still have their dark brown coating.
- Potatoes should not be washed before storage nor refrigerated; storing them at temperatures below 40 to 50°F can convert some of the starch to sugar.

- Sweets eaten between meals can be more damaging to teeth than those eaten with meals.
- Honey can cause botulism in infants because of their undeveloped digestive systems.
- Anticoagulant (blood-thinning) medications can be dangerously undermined by daily consumption of such vitamin K–rich foods as cabbage, lettuce, asparagus, turnip greens, and spinach.
- Comfrey tea, used frequently to soothe stomachs and alleviate ulcer pain, contains cancer-causing alkaloids.
- Taking antibiotics too soon after—or not long enough before—meals can prevent them from reaching adequate levels of effectiveness to cure the disease or infection for which they have been prescribed.
- Pasta packaged in containers with a clear viewing window can lose up to half of its riboflavin in twenty-four hours at room temperature.
- Heavy consumption of soybeans can reduce the effectiveness of thyroid medications.
- A diet *too* high in fiber-rich foods can interfere with your body's ability to use calcium, magnesium, iron, and zinc.

## 143. International Cuisine Kudos and Cautions

Many foreign foods have been found to offer amazing health benefits. For example:

- Japanese miso soup, made from fermented soybeans and grains, seems to reduce stomach cancer.
- Indian yogurt is a natural antibiotic that has been helpful in lowering cholesterol levels and in the treatment of hepatitis, gallstones, and kidney disorders.
- Italian olive oil is highly monounsaturated and has been shown to surpass all polyunsaturated oils in helping to prevent heart disease.
- Mexican corn and beans provide low-fat, high-fiber protein with large amounts of calcium (the corn is steeped in limewater) and other nutrients, and chili peppers have been found helpful in

fighting asthma, bronchitis, and sinusitis. (The American Heart Association recommends salsa as a low-salt condiment.)

- Chinese mushrooms, particularly shiitake and enoki mushrooms, appear to contain powerful stimulators of the immune system.

But even the best international cuisines have their nutritional drawbacks. And when you are eating out, they should definitely be kept in mind.

**INDIAN FOOD** Steer clear of dishes that are drenched in ghee.

**JAPANESE FOOD** Watch out for smoked foods, which are high in nitrates, and dishes cooked with large amounts of high-sodium soy sauce.

**ITALIAN FOOD** Beware of pasta smothered in rich cheese, cream, and butter sauces.

**MEXICAN FOOD** Keep away from commercially prepared refried beans that are usually made with lard.

**CHINESE FOOD** Soups can be hazardous since they're almost always prepared beforehand and laden with MSG. Also, adding extra soy sauce to any dish is dangerous since most are already prepared with this high-sodium condiment.

## 144. A Not-for-Seniors Reminder

Seniors—and others who face special risks of illness, such as pregnant women, children, and people with compromised immune systems—are advised not to eat:

- Raw fin fish and shellfish, including oysters, clams, scallops, and mussels.
- Soft cheeses such as Brie, feta, Camembert, blue-veined, and Mexican-style cheese.
- Raw or lightly cooked egg products including salad dressings, and cookie or cake batter.
- Raw meat or poultry.
- Raw sprouts.
- Unpasteurized or untreated milk, cheese, or fruit or vegetable juices.

## 145. Do You Know the Foods That Supply Your Nutrients?

### A QUICK VITAMIN, MINERAL, AND
### AMINO ACID REFERENCE LIST

| Vitamin | Best Natural Sources |
| --- | --- |
| Vitamin A | Fish-liver oil, liver, carrots, green and yellow vegetables, eggs, milk and dairy products, margarine, yellow fruits |
| Vitamin $B_1$ (thiamine) | Dried yeast, rice husks, whole wheat, oatmeal, peanuts, pork, most vegetables, bran, milk |
| Vitamin $B_2$ (riboflavin) | Milk, liver, kidney, yeast, cheese, leafy green vegetables, fish, eggs |
| Vitamin $B_6$ (pyridoxine) | Brewer's yeast, wheat bran, wheat germ, liver, kidney, heart, cantaloupe, cabbage, blackstrap molasses, milk, eggs, beef |
| Vitamin $B_{12}$ (cobalamin) | Liver, beef, pork, eggs, milk, cheese, kidney |
| Vitamin $B_{12}$ (orotic acid) | Root vegetables, whey (the liquid portion of soured or curdled milk) |
| Vitamin $B_{15}$ (pangamic acid) | Brewer's yeast, whole brown rice, whole grains, pumpkin seeds, sesame seeds |
| Vitamin $B_{17}$ (laetrile) | A small amount of laetrile is found in the whole kernels of apricots, apples, cherries, peaches, plums, and nectarines. |
| Biotin (coenzyme R or vitamin H) | Nuts, fruits, brewer's yeast, beef liver, milk, kidney, unpolished rice |
| Vitamin C (ascorbic acid) | Citrus fruits, berries, green leafy vegetables, tomatoes, cauliflower, potatoes, sweet potatoes |

| Vitamin | Best Natural Sources |
|---|---|
| Calcium pantothenate (pantothenic acid, pantothenol, vitamin $B_5$) | Meat, whole grains, wheat germ, bran, kidney, liver, heart, green leafy vegetables, brewer's yeast, nuts, chicken, crude molasses |
| Choline | Egg yolk, brain, heart, green leafy vegetables, yeast liver, wheat germ (and, in small amounts, in lecithin) |
| Vitamin D (calciferol, viosterol, ergosterol) | Wheat germ, soybeans, vegetable oils, broccoli, brussels sprouts, leafy greens, spinach, enriched flour, whole wheat, whole-grain cereals, eggs |
| Vitamin E (tocopherol) | Wheat germ, soybeans, vegetable oils, broccoli, brussels sprouts, leafy greens, spinach, enriched flour, whole wheat, whole-grain cereals, eggs |
| Vitamin F (unsaturated fatty acids: linoleic, linolenic, and arachidonic) | Vegetable oils (wheat germ, linseed, sunflower, safflower, soybean, and peanut), peanuts, sunflower seeds, walnuts, pecans, almonds, avocados |
| Folic acid (folacin) | Deep green leafy vegetables, carrots, tortula yeast, liver, egg yolk, cantaloupe, apricots, pumpkins, avocados, beans, whole-wheat and dark rye flour |
| Inositol | Liver, brewer's yeast, dried lima beans, beef brains and heart, cantaloupe, grapefruit, raisins, wheat germ, unrefined molasses, peanuts, cabbage |
| Vitamin K (menadione) | Yogurt, alfalfa, egg yolk, safflower oil, soybean oil, fish-liver oils, kelp, leafy green vegetables |

| Vitamin | Best Natural Sources |
|---|---|
| Niacin (nicotinic acid, niacinamide, nicotinamide) | Liver, lean meat, whole-wheat products, brewer's yeast, kidney, wheat germ, fish, eggs, roasted peanuts, the white meat of poultry, avocados, dates, figs, prunes |
| Vitamin P (C complex, citrus bioflavonoids, rutin, hesperidin) | The white skin and segment part of citrus fruit (lemons, oranges, grapefruit); also in apricots, buckwheat, blackberries, cherries, rose hips |
| PABA (para-aminobenzoic acid) | Liver, brewer's yeast, kidney, whole grains, rice, bran, wheat germ, molasses |

| Mineral | Best Natural Sources |
|---|---|
| Calcium | Milk, milk products, all cheeses, soybeans, sardines, salmon, peanuts, sunflower seeds, dried beans, green vegetables |
| Chlorine | Table salt, kelp, olives |
| Chromium | Meat, shellfish, chicken, corn oil, clams, brewer's yeast |
| Cobalt | Milk, kidney, liver, red meat, oysters, clams |
| Copper | Dried beans, peas, whole wheat, prunes, liver, shrimp, and most other seafood |
| Fluorine | Seafood and gelatin |
| Iodine (Iodide) | Kelp, vegetables grown in iodine-rich soil, onions, all seafood |
| Iron | Pork liver, beef kidney, heart, and liver, farina, raw clams, dried peaches, red meat, egg yolk, oysters, nuts, beans, asparagus, molasses, oatmeal |

| Mineral | Best Natural Sources |
|---|---|
| Magnesium | Figs, lemons, grapefruit, yellow corn, almonds, nuts, seeds, dark green leafy vegetables, apples |
| Manganese | Nuts, green leafy vegetables, peas, beets, egg yolk, whole-grain cereals |
| Molybdenum | Dark green leafy vegetables, whole grains, eggs, nuts, seeds |
| Phosphorus | Fish, poultry, meat, whole grains, eggs, nuts, seeds |
| Potassium | Citrus fruits, watercress, green leafy vegetables, mint leaves, sunflower seeds, bananas, potatoes |
| Selenium | Wheat germ, bran, tuna fish, onions, tomatoes, broccoli |
| Sodium | Salt, shellfish, carrots, beets, artichokes, dried beef, brains, kidney, bacon |
| Sulfur | Lean beef, dried beans, fish, eggs, cabbage |
| Vanadium | Fish |
| Water | Drinking water, juices, fruits, vegetables |
| Zinc | Round steak, lamb chops, pork loin, wheat germ, brewer's yeast, pumpkin seeds, eggs, nonfat dry milk, ground mustard |

| Amino Acids | Best Natural Sources |
|---|---|
| Tryptophan | Cottage cheese, milk, turkey, bananas, meat, dried dates, peanuts, all protein-rich foods |

| Amino Acids | Best Natural Sources |
|---|---|
| Phenylalanine | Soy products, bread stuffing, cottage cheese, nonfat dry milk, almonds, peanuts, lima beans, pumpkin seeds, sesame seeds, all protein-rich foods |
| Lysine | Fish, milk, lima beans, meat, cheese, yeast, eggs, soy products, all protein-rich foods |
| Arginine | Nuts, popcorn, carob, gelatin desserts, chocolate, brown rice, oatmeal, raisins, sunflower and sesame seeds, whole-wheat bread, all protein-rich foods |

# 146. Any Questions About Chapter 11?

*If mayonnaise spoils so easily, why is it never refrigerated in the supermarket?*

Mayonnaise doesn't spoil easily. In fact, unopened and unrefrigerated, it can remain fresh for at least six months, usually longer. Despite all the concern about food poisoning at picnics, mayonnaise is seldom, if ever, the cause. (It's too acidic for bacteria to grow in easily.) What happens is that when it is mixed with other foods, such as tuna fish, eggs, and potatoes, it becomes a medium for bacterial growth.

The reason manufacturers recommend that it be refrigerated after opening is because when adding it to salads, most people will dip in for another spoonful, leaving some particles of food that can cause it to become a bacterial breeding ground. If kept refrigerated at temperatures of 40°F, it will remain harmless. Salads mixed with mayonnaise should be kept cold until ready to eat. Leaving them out for hours gives bacteria a field day and picnickers the trots.

*Is it safe to refreeze foods that have only partially thawed?*

If the foods still contain ice crystals and have been held no longer than one or two days at refrigerator temperatures after thawing, they're generally safe to refreeze. (Thawed ice cream is an exception; it should not be refrozen.) As a rule, if a partially thawed food is safe to eat, it's safe to refreeze, although nutritional quality may be reduced. On the other hand, if there are any off odors or colors, the food should definitely not be refrozen or eaten.

*When I was recovering from a nasty case of food poisoning, my doctor prescribed carrot soup. I was surprised. Has chicken soup been nutritionally usurped for some reason?*

Not at all. Chicken soup is, and probably always will be, "Jewish penicillin" because of its natural antibiotic properties. But when recovering from dehydration caused by diarrhea, which you undoubtedly were, sodium and potassium are the two electrolytes most needed to be returned in proper balance. And carrot soup has them—in the correct proportions. According to Dr. Jan Soule, the Portland, Oregon, pediatrician who dished out the information to the medical community as well as to his patients, carrot soup is one of the best rehydrators.

Bouillon and canned soups have far too much sodium, and juices, although high in potassium, haven't a balanced amount of sodium. Herb teas can replace lost water but not electrolytes, and caffeinated beverages can *promote* dehydration. The soup can be made in a jiffy by combining equal amounts of water and commercial strained baby carrots (which have salt in them) and bringing the mixture to a boil.

*I'm pregnant and my doctor told me I shouldn't eat smoked fish. I don't understand why it's a health risk.*

There have been outbreaks of listeriosis linked to the consumption of smoked fish. It is not the temperature reached during the smoking that affects the bacterial count, but the length of time the fish has been smoked. Since you've no way of knowing if the fish has been smoked for the safe level of at least twelve hours, it's best to avoid it. Chemotherapy patients, and anyone with AIDS or other immune-system disease, should also avoid it.

# FOOD FOR THOUGHT

- Believe it or not, it's true! According to the USDA Meat and Poultry Hotline it is *not necessary* to rinse chicken and fish before cooking. The more you handle these foods, the greater the chance that organisms on them will be transferred to your hands and other foods. Proper cooking will kill any surface bacteria on raw food. Always wash hands thoroughly with hot soapy water after touching raw meat, fish, or poultry.
- At room temperature, bacteria in food can double every twenty minutes!
- Dirty dishes left to soak in the sink create an unhealthy soup. According to Robert Buchanan, Ph.D., food safety initiative lead scientist in the Food and Drug Administration's Center for Food Safety and Applied Nutrition, the food left on the dishes contributes nutrients for bacteria, and the bacteria multiply. If washing dishes by hand, it's best to wash them all within two hours—and air-dry them so you don't handle them while they're wet.

Chapter Twelve

# The Disease and Wellness Connection

## 147. The Diet–Disease Link

The evidence linking diet to cancer, heart disease, diabetes, infertility, depression, and numerous other ailments is becoming stronger and stronger. Researchers are finding that overconsumption of foods high in fats and additives—unchecked by those high in fiber, anticarcinogens, and essential nutrients—can cause diseases that are far easier to prevent than cure.

This does not mean that any one diet, or particular food or supplement regimen, is the answer. Despite all the books and articles you might have read or heard about, *no diet can guarantee protection against illness.* But learning what foods have been shown to contribute to certain illnesses, avoiding or limiting their consumption, and counteracting their risks with alternative health-boosting foods and a supplement regimen to cover your nutritional bases (see section 31) can provide you with the best chance for a longer and healthier life.

## 148. Cancer Brewers

The National Academy of Sciences, National Cancer Institute, and American Cancer Society recommend that no more than 20 to 30 percent of the calories in your diet come from fat. Individuals whose diets contain over 40 percent fat, saturated as well as unsaturated, are more likely to develop colon, breast, and prostate cancers.

The following percentages of calories from fat, compiled by the Center of Science in the Public Interest, are given here to alert you to frequently eaten foods that you might want to eat less of. For example, 2 tablespoons of mayonnaise have only 200 calories, but because 100 percent of those calories are fat, those 2 tablespoons equal 34 percent of your daily calorie intake, in effect more than *half* of what is considered a safe daily fat allotment. (If you're not up to dividing the number of calories in your food portions by their fat percentages, see section 104.)

| FOOD | CALORIES FROM FAT |
| --- | --- |
| Butter, margarine, mayonnaise, oils | 100 percent |
| Coconut | 92 percent |
| Cream cheese | 90 percent |
| Avocado | 86 percent |
| Beef franks, bologna | 80 percent |
| Peanut butter | 76 percent |
| Cheddar cheese | 74 percent |
| Chicken franks | 68 percent |
| Swiss cheese | 66 percent |
| Ground beef (lean) | 65 percent |
| Eggs, potato chips | 63 percent |
| Croissant (Pepperidge Farm) | 59 percent |
| Mozzarella cheese (part skim), chicken breast (Kentucky Fried), milk chocolate candy bars | 56 percent |
| Old-fashioned doughnuts (Hostess), Big Mac (McDonald's) | 53 percent |

| FOOD | CALORIES FROM FAT |
|---|---|
| Ricotta cheese (part skim), tofu, Fillet-o-Fish (McDonald's) | 52 percent |
| Pork chop (lean), hamburger (Wendy's) | 50 percent |
| Whole milk (4 percent fat) | 49 percent |
| Vanilla ice cream | 48 percent |
| French fries | 47 percent |
| Stouffer's entrées (average) | 46 percent |
| Le Menu and Armour Dinner Classics (average), lamb (rib chop), veal (round) | 45 percent |
| Chicken (dark, w/out skin) | 43 percent |
| Apple pie (Morton's) | 40 percent |
| Cottage cheese (4 percent fat) | 39 percent |
| Low-fat milk (2 percent), hamburger (McDonald's) | 38 percent |
| Granola cereals | 32–42 percent |
| Round steak (lean) | 29 percent |
| Chicken (light, w/out skin) | 24 percent |
| Low-fat milk (1 percent) | 23 percent |
| Yogurt (low-fat, plain) | 22 percent |
| Lean Cuisine meals (average) | 21 percent |

## OTHER EDIBLE CANCER CONCERNS

- Food additives, particularly BHA, BHT, FD&C Red No. 3, Blue No. 2, Green No. 3, and Citrus Red No. 2, propyl gallate, and sodium nitrite
- Coffee, regular or decaffeinated (implicated in bladder and pancreatic cancers)
- Liver and high-fat fish, such as bluefish, striped bass, lake trout, and mackerel; and bottom-feeding fish, such as carp, which are more likely than others to contain high levels of contaminants
- Alcohol (found to cause liver cancer and contribute to cancers of the mouth, throat, larynx, and esophagus, particularly among smokers)

## 149. Foods That Can Fight Back

Foods high in vitamins A, C, and E, selenium, and fiber (see section 145) have been found to help in the prevention of cancer. Eating three or more ½-cup servings of vegetables daily, particularly those rich in beta-carotene and cruciferous vegetables containing indoles and isothiocyanates (substances that have been found to reduce the number of tumors in mice treated with carcinogens) is highly recommended.

Cruciferous vegetables that have been found to contain indoles and isothiocyanates are broccoli, brussels sprouts, cabbage, and cauliflower. Other cruciferous vegetables that are presumed to contain indoles and isothiocyanates include bok choy, collards, kale, kohlrabi, mustard greens, rutabaga, and turnips.

Foods rich in beta-carotene are carrots, cantaloupe, squash, papaya, and sweet potatoes.

Quercetin, which may suppress malignant cells before they become tumors, is found in onions (and not destroyed by cooking).

Foods rich in omega-3 fatty acids, such as salmon, tuna, and sardines, help the immune system prevent and inhibit spreading cancers.

And don't forget soybeans and soy-based foods, which are high in many cancer-fighting phytochemicals. (See section 109.)

## 150. Food Mood Swingers

There's little doubt that what we eat affects how we feel. In fact, numerous experiments have proven that many symptoms of mental illness can be switched off and on by changing the diet and altering nutrient levels in the body.

| NUTRIENT | WHAT IT CAN DO |
| --- | --- |
| Vitamin $B_1$ (thiamine) | Large amounts have been found to tranquilize anxious individuals and alleviate depression. |
| Vitamin $B_2$ (riboflavin) | Works synergistically with vitamins $B_6$ and C, and niacin as a stress fighter. |

|  |  |
|---|---|
|  | Insufficiencies are frequently found in individuals whose diets are too low in meat or dairy protein. |
| Vitamin B$_6$ (pyridoxine) | Insufficiencies can impair the function of the adrenal cortex and adversely affect production of natural anti-depressants such as dopamine and norepinephrine. |
| Choline | One of the few nutrients able to penetrate the blood–brain barrier, which ordinarily protects the brain against variations in the daily diet, and go directly into brain cells to produce a chemical that aids memory. Dietary insufficiencies are frequently manifest by nervousness or twitching. |
| Pantothenic acid | A natural tension reliever when sufficient in the diet. |
| Vitamin C (ascorbic acid) | Needed along with vitamin B$_6$ for the effective conversion of phenylalanine into mood-elevating norepinephrine. |
| Vitamin B$_{12}$ (cobalamin) | Insufficient amounts can impair concentration, promote irritability, decrease energy, and increase anxiety. |
| Vitamin E (alpha-tocopherol) | Important for supplying adequate oxygen to brain cells. |
| Folic acid (folacin) | Deficiencies have been found to be contributing factors in mental illness. |
| Zinc | Promotes mental alertness and aids in proper brain function; deficiencies have frequently been found in schizophrenics. |

| NUTRIENT | WHAT IT CAN DO |
|---|---|
| Magnesium | Necessary for healthy nerve functioning; known as the antistress mineral. |
| Niacin | Lack of this B-complex vitamin can bring out negative personality changes. |
| Calcium | Alleviates tension and irritability, and promotes relaxation. |
| Tyrosine | An amino acid that releases a substance called catecholamine, which, in turn, increases the production of the antidepressants dopamine and norepinephrine. |
| Tryptophan | An amino acid that functions synergistically with vitamin $B_6$, niacin, and magnesium to synthesize serotonin, a natural tranquilizer. (The availability of tryptophan and tyrosine in the brain is a major factor in determining the rate at which vital neurotransmitters are produced; within one hour after a meal moods can change according to the rise and fall of these two amino acids in the blood.) |
| Phenylalanine | An essential amino acid (found in cheese, meat, milk, and eggs) necessary for the manufacture and release of the brain's antidepressants dopamine and norepinephrine. |

## 151. Eating Your Way to Depression

The quickest way to ruin your day is by eating the wrong food. Refined sugars and carbohydrates (particularly those in cookies, potato chips, pretzels, sugared cereals, and junk foods) deplete your body of mood-regulating nutrients. Moreover, they play Ping-Pong with your glucose levels to the point of promoting antisocial, aggressive, and often violent behavior. (It has been found that 75 percent of all criminals have abnormal glucose levels.)

- Children and adolescents on high-sugar, refined-carbohydrate diets have been found to undergo personality changes.
- Regular consumption of processed luncheon meats (bologna, hot dogs, ham, and so on) or convenience foods with artificial colorings and other additives can not only deplete essential stress-fighting B vitamins and zinc, but cause allergic reactions as well. (In children, these may cause a chemical reaction in the brain that's manifested by a sudden outburst of delinquent behavior.)
- If you are allergic to gluten, consuming products containing wheat, oats, rye, barley, or vegetables such as beans, cabbage, turnips, dried peas, and cucumbers can cause depression and fatigue. The same holds true if you are allergic to, and deliberately or inadvertently consume, dairy or citrus products.
- Chocolate, cocoa, and all caffeine-containing beverages (see section 61) can inhibit the proper assimilation of calcium and deplete the body of B-complex vitamins and zinc.
- Alcohol from wine, beer, spirits, or cough syrups can rob the body of vitamins $B_1$ and $B_2$, choline, niacin, folic acid, and magnesium.

## 152. Depression and Stress Antidotes

**APPETIZING UPPERS**

Whole-wheat products, brewer's yeast, wheat germ, fish, eggs, peanuts, the white meat of poultry, avocados, dates, figs, prunes, rice husks, oatmeal, bran, milk, green leafy vegetables, cantaloupe, cabbage, blackstrap molasses, lean meat, cheese, citrus fruits, berries, tomatoes, cauliflower, broccoli, brussels sprouts, ground mustard, potatoes, sweet potatoes, soybeans, sardines, salmon, walnuts, sunflower seeds, dried beans, dairy products, yellow corn, almonds, apples, lemons, grapefruit, peas, beets, bananas, lima beans, pumpkin seeds, and sesame seeds

## DELICIOUS DESTRESSORS

- A glass of warm milk before bedtime is a soothing source of tryptophan, and can reduce anxiety and tension.
- Celery juice is a tangy and effective nerve unjangler for weight-conscious working men and women.
- A high-carbohydrate dinner can help you unwind and relax by raising the level of serotonin in the brain.

(**Note:** Because stress speeds up potassium loss, be sure to include bananas, potatoes, citrus fruits, and other potassium-rich foods in your daily diet.)

## 153. Foods Can Be Sex Sinkers

Just because you or your partner is not in the mood for love as often as you'd like to be doesn't necessarily mean that something is missing in your relationship. It could be missing from your diet.

A deficiency in zinc can cause a definite diminution of your sex drive. Vegetarians might make lousy lovers if they are consuming excessive amounts of calcium-rich greens and whole-grain cereals, breads, and bran, which contain phytic acid, because high intakes of these can prevent the absorption of zinc.

Drinking large amounts of coffee or other caffeinated beverages might keep you awake but put your sexual urges to sleep by inhibiting zinc absorption.

Eating frequent and hefty amounts of ice cream, beverages, candy, baked goods, gelatin desserts, and chewing gums that are artificially flavored with benzyl alcohol, butyl acetate, or benzaldehyde can produce central nervous system depression and reduce sexual urges and pleasures to memories.

If you are planning on having a family, avoid frequent consumption of shortening, processed breakfast cereals, instant potatoes, snack foods, and others containing propyl gallate. This antioxidant has been implicated as a cause of reproductive failures.

Cocktails for two are romantic, but more than two cocktails can turn one enchanted evening into another depressing washout. Alcohol might increase sexual desire, but as many drinkers have discovered, that's about all it increases.

## 154. Great Boosters for Better Sex

### LOVE ENERGIZERS

Oysters, wheat germ, pumpkin and sunflower seeds, seafood, poultry, soybeans, melon, meat, avocados, green leafy vegetables, olive oil, eggs, whole-grain cereals, low-fat milk

### HERBS WITH SEX APPEAL

- Sarsaparilla has been used as a natural sexual stimulant for centuries. (The sarsaparilla plant has chemical substances with testosterone, progesterone, and cortisol activity, which probably accounts for its usefulness in increasing sexual appetites.) It is best when prepared by boiling an ounce of sarsaparilla root in a pint of water for half an hour and most effective if wine-size (4- to 6-ounce) glassfuls of it are drunk regularly.
- Damiana, an herb that's also called turnea, is known as a natural aphrodisiac. By simply pouring a cup of boiling water over a teaspoonful of the dried leaves (or ¼ teaspoonful of the ground leaf powder), it can be made into tea. Drinking 1 to 4 cups daily (no more) has provided some tantalizing rewards for many who've tried it.
- Because of its normalizing effect on the body's metabolism, ginseng (see section 132) drunk as a tea or tonic can help reduce anxiety and heighten sexual stimulation.

## 155. Aging Accelerators

Everyone knows that eating the wrong foods in the wrong quantities can increase weight rapidly. But everyone doesn't know that it can also accelerate aging.

- Coffee, tea, cocoa, colas, and other caffeinated beverages are liquid youth-liquidators that dehydrate your skin and can cause premature wrinkling.
- Diet sodas with aspartame may diminish brain function. Aspartic acid is an "excitotoxin" because it overstimulates neurons, which eventually burn out.
- There's no harm in an occasional glass of wine, but immoderate alcohol consumption can dehydrate skin, dilate blood vessels, foster spidery broken capillaries on the face, and add years to your looks while subtracting them from your life. (See section 90.)
- High-fat, high-protein, low-carbohydrate diets—or any liquid, fad, or crash reducing programs that produce a rapid weight loss by eliminating a category of nutrients—are dangerous promoters of aging. Aside from causing skin to lose elasticity, and depleting nutrients necessary for the healthy regeneration of cells, they engender stress that can cause the release of actual aging chemicals in the body.
- Meat and milk, if consumed in large quantities, can inhibit the absorption of manganese, which is essential for the production of the antiaging enzyme SOD (superoxide dismutase). SOD, which diminishes naturally as we age, fortifies the body against the ravages of free radicals, the destructive molecules that speed the aging process by destroying healthy cells and collagen.
- Processed foods that are high in refined carbohydrates and sugar can contribute to vision problems.
- Too much salt in the diet may cause more calcium to be excreted in the urine and increase the risk of osteoporosis.
- Excessive consumption of soft drinks, which are high in phosphorus, can also deplete you of calcium and increase your chances of osteoporosis.

## 156. Help for Holding Back Advancing Years

**YOUTH EXTENDERS**

Wheat germ, bran, whole grains, spinach, asparagus, mushrooms, fish (especially sardines, salmon, and mackerel), chicken liver, oatmeal, onions, pumpkin seeds, brewer's yeast, dried beans, peas, prunes, green leafy vegetables, low-fat milk, olive oil

**VICTUALS FOR VITALITY**

- A fish dish a day (or at least five times weekly) can help your body stay well supplied with the DNA–RNA nucleic acids that are essential for new cell growth.
- Eating substantial amounts of foods rich in PABA and folic acid (see section 145) can help retard the graying of hair and possibly even return gray hair to its former color.
- An orange, a 1-ounce slice of cheddar cheese, and a glass of skim milk can supply half of your daily requirement for calcium—a pretty simple way to help keep your skin smooth, bones strong, and nerves on a healthy even keel.

## 157. Immunity Underminers

A healthy immune system is a stalwart army of white blood cells (called T-cells because they're controlled by the thymus gland) that is instructed where and when to attack and what antibiotics their cofighters (called B-cells because they're made in the bone marrow) should produce. As you get older your thymus gland decreases in power and size, becomes a less effective commander of your defense brigade, and if not supplied with the right nutritional reinforcements, will let you down—the hard way.

Highly allergenic foods, such as shellfish, chocolate, and eggs, can cause the immune systems of susceptible individuals to create excessive antibodies when none are needed, resulting in a variety of discomforting and potentially dangerous symptoms.

- Frequent consumption of foods containing artificial flavors, colors, MSG, and other additives can stress the immune system, diminishing its effectiveness in protecting you from numerous illnesses and infections.
- Indulging in refined carbohydrates (cakes, cookies, junk food, and so on), caffeine, and alcohol can make you more vulnerable to infection and illness by depleting essential immune system nutrients.
- Irradiated foods, eaten on a regular basis, may impair bone marrow and adversely affect the immune system's production of B-cells.

## 158. Boosting Your Body's Defenses

### THE NATURAL "RAMBOS"

Carrots, fish (sardines, salmon, mackerel), skim milk, citrus fruits, green leafy vegetables, wheat germ, whole grains, bran, soybeans, broccoli, brussels sprouts, eggs, sesame seeds, brown rice, nuts, onions, pumpkin seeds, ground mustard, brewer's yeast, propolis, papaya

### THE RIGHT FUEL

- A diet low in fat and high in complex carbohydrates, especially those that are rich in fiber, will strengthen the immune system.
- Evening primrose oil, an herb containing the active ingredient gamma linoleic acid (GLA), can help in the production of hormonelike compounds called prostaglandins—which are vital to the immune system.
- Propolis, a resinlike material found in leaf buds and the bark of trees and collected by bees whose enzymes convert it into pollen, is a thymus gland stimulator and natural immune system enhancer.

## 159. Any Questions About Chapter 12?

*I'm forty years old and my face still breaks out. I am a vegetarian, and I don't drink, smoke, or eat junk food. I eat only natural foods, lots of grains, and I can't imagine what in my diet is causing this.*

It could be any of a number of things. It could even *be* a number of things—hormonal changes, allergic reaction, stress, and so on—but if it is diet related, I'd suspect it is being caused by some androgenic (rich in male hormones) food. You might try keeping away from peanuts, peanut oil, wheat germ oil, and brewer's yeast for a while and see if your skin clears up. The amount of male hormones in these foods is small, but for anyone with a latent skin or hair problem, it's enough to cause trouble.

*I've been on a very healthy and successful diet for the past four months (high fiber, low fat) and have lost 32 pounds. I feel fine, except for the fact that I haven't menstruated since I began dieting. I take a supplement daily, eat salad twice a day. My gynecologist found nothing wrong with me. What could I be missing?*

My guess would be calories. The physical stress of losing more than 30 pounds (or as much as 15 percent of your body weight) in a relatively short time can suppress production of hypothalamic and pituitary hormones that are essential to the menstrual cycle. If you are exercising, you might be overdoing it. Keep in mind that diets providing fewer than 1,200 calories daily can cause problems and should not be undertaken without the supervision of a doctor. I'd advise eating 300 to 500 more calories daily and easing up on your workouts. If you don't start menstruating within four weeks, it's time for another visit to the gynecologist.

*I've been told that there's an herb now on the market that can help cure impotence. Do you know anything about it?*

There are several herbs that say they can help cure impotence. Yohimbine, an extract of the bark of the yohimbe tree, has been used as a treatment, but it is potentially toxic to the liver, can cause a sudden decline in blood pressure, and should only be used under the direction of a doctor. However, the herb damiana is a tonic for the sex organs and is safe to take. The usual dose is up to three capsules daily. Other than that, I suggest ginkgo biloba, 60 mg three times daily; two to four saw palmetto–zinc–pumpkin seed oil combination capsules daily; and arginine, 4 to 5 g, taken forty-five minutes before sex.

## FOOD FOR THOUGHT

- A ten-year study conducted by the University of Bristol, England, found that men who have sex three or more times a week reduce their risk of a major heart attack or stroke by about 50 percent!
- Almost 20 percent of people older than age sixty-five have diabetes. Type 2 diabetes, often caused by obesity, accounts for 90 to 95 percent of these cases. Type 2 diabetes reduces the life expectancy of middle-aged people by five to ten years and is undiagnosed in 10 to 15 percent of people over the age of fifty. Additionally, people with diabetes are about twice as likely to have arteriosclerosis or ischemic heart disease and are two and a half times more likely to have a stroke than people without diabetes.
- People who spend four hours or more a day in front of the TV are twice as likely to be overweight. If you watch two hours a day, you're 57 percent more likely to be overweight than those who keep tube time to an hour or less.

# Chapter Thirteen

# May I Help You?

### 160. How to Locate a Nutritionally Oriented Doctor

If you would like to consult a nutritionally oriented physician—or other alternative health practitioner—but don't know any in your area, the following organizations may be able to help you find one. You should specify if you're seeking a board certified physician, as not all nutritional health professionals are M.D.s.

Organizations that have home pages on the World Wide Web—and most do—can provide you with immediate information about licensing, certification, and the fastest way to access a local practitioner. (If you are not online, you can probably find a library in your area that is.)

*It should be understood that no endorsement or other opinion of any practitioner contacted through these services (or such practitioner's diagnoses, treatments, or credentials) is implied or should be inferred.*

(If you contact an organization by mail, as a courtesy please enclose a self-addressed, stamped envelope with all queries.)

## RESOURCES

### American Academy of Medical Acupuncture (AAMA)
5820 Wilshire Blvd., Suite 500
Los Angeles, CA 90036
(213) 937-5514 or 1-800-521-2262
Web site: www.medicalacupuncture.org

### American Academy of Osteopathy (AAO)
3500 DePauw Blvd., Suite 1080
Indianapolis, IN 46268
(317) 879-1881
Web site: www.aao.medguide.net

### American Association of Naturopathic Physicians
601 Valley, Suite 105
Seattle, WA 98109
(206) 298-0126 or (206) 298-0125 (referral line)
Web site: www.naturopathic.org

### American Chiropractic Association (ACA)
1701 Clarendon Blvd., Suite 200
Arlington, VA 22209
(703) 276-8800 or 1-800-986-4646
Web site: www.amerchiro.org

### American Holistic Medical Association
6728 Old McLean Village Drive
McLean, VA 22101
(703) 556-9728
Web site: www.ahma.holistic.com

### American Holistic Nurses Association
P.O. Box 2130
Flagstaff, AZ 86003-2130
1-800-278-2462 or 1-800-278-AHNA
Web site: www.ahna.org

**Council for Responsible Nutrition**
1875 Eye St., NW, Suite 400
Washington, DC 20006
(202) 872-1488
Web site: www.crnusa.org

**Homeopathic Academy of Naturopathic Physicians (HANP)**
1232 South East Foster Place
Portland, OR 97266
(503) 761-3298; Fax: (503) 762-1929
Web site: www.healthy.net/hanp

**National Center for Complementary and Alternative Medicine (NCCAM) at the National Institutes of Health (NIH)**
NCCAM Clearinghouse
P.O. Box 7923
Gaithersburg, MD 20898
1-888-644-6226; Fax: 1-866-464-3616
Web site: www.nccam.nih.gov

**National Center for Homeopathy**
801 N. Fairfax, Suite 306
Alexandria, VA 22314
(703) 548-7790; Fax: (703) 548-7792
Web site: www.homeopathic.org

**Practitioners of Alternative Medicine USA & World**
Web site: www.sonic.net/~nexus/listdocs.html

## 161. Free Calls for Fast Answers

- For information about diet and cancer, the National Cancer Institute will answer any question it can. Just call 1-800-4-Cancer.
- For information on water contaminants, waste-disposal sites, and dangerous chemicals, the Environmental Protection Agency's hotline is 1-800-546-8740.

- For product recall information, the Consumer Product Safety Commission's hotline is 1-800-638-2772.
- To register complaints about food fraud, waste, or abuse, call the Department of Agriculture's hotline, 1-800-535-4555.
- For answers to questions about the safety of your drinking water, you can phone the EPA Safe Drinking Water Hotline, 1-800-426-4791.
- For information on health and safety of baby foods, contact the Gerber hotline at 1-800-4 GERBER.
- If you want to know more about herbs, where to obtain them, and have questions about their safety and usage, you can call Green Mountain Herbs (1-800-525-2696), or Foodscience Corporation (1-800-451-5190) for the answers.
- Vegetarians who would like to learn more ways to use meat analogs in their diets can call Morningstar Farms, a division of Miles Laboratories, for recipes and suppliers. The toll-free number is 1-800-243-4143.

# Afterword

I HOPE I'VE been able to provide enough information to enable you to minimize the risks of foods and maximize their potential for providing you with health, longevity, and happiness at every meal.

With that in mind, I leave you with these parting morsels:

- Heptachlor, a carcinogenic grain pesticide banned in 1988, is still showing up in mother's breast milk.
- Every unwanted nutrient in the American diet is supplied in large doses by white bread, rolls, and crackers, because they're eaten so frequently.
- Some of us may live to eat, but all of us must eat to live—and what we eat *can* change our lives.

To your health!
EARL L. MINDELL, R.PH., PH.D.
Beverly Hills, California
November 2001

# Glossary

**Absorption**  The process by which nutrients are passed into the bloodstream.

**Acetate**  A derivative of acetic acid.

**Acetic acid**  Used as a synthetic flavoring agent, one of the first food additives (vinegar is approximately 4 to 6 percent acetic acid); it is found naturally in cheese, coffee, grapes, peaches, raspberries, and strawberries.

**Acetone**  A colorless solvent for fat, oils, and waxes that is obtained by fermentation (inhalation can irritate the lungs, and large amounts have a narcotic effect).

**Acid**  A water-soluble substance with a sour taste.

**Addiction**  Compulsive use of a habit-forming substance.

**Adrenal gland**  A triangular-shaped gland near each kidney that synthesizes and stores dopamine, norepinephrine, and epinephrine.

**Alkali**  An acid-neutralizing substance (sodium bicarbonate is alkali used for excess acidity in foods).

**Allergen**  A substance that causes an allergy.

**Allergy**  Abnormal sensitivity to any substance.

**Amenorrhea**  Absence or suppression of menstruation.

**Amino acid chelates**  Chelated minerals that have been produced by many of the same processes nature uses to chelate minerals in the body in the digestive tract, permitting them to be absorbed into the bloodstream.

**Amino acids**  The organic compounds from which proteins are constructed; there are twenty-three known amino acids, but only nine are indispensable nutrients for humans—histidine, isoleucine, leucine, lysine, total S-containing amino acids, total aromatic amino acids, threonine, tryptophan, and valine—and must be obtained from food.

**Analgesic**  Drug used to relieve pain.

**Anemia**  Reduction in normal amount of red blood cells.

**Anorectic**  Having no appetite.

**Anorexia nervosa**  A mental disturbance that causes loss of appetite for food and compulsive dieting.

**Antibiotic**  Any of various substances that are effective in inhibiting or destroying bacteria.

**Anticoagulant**  Something that delays or prevents blood clotting; blood thinner.

**Antidyskinetics**  Drugs used in the treatment of Parkinson's disease.

**Antiemetic**  Remedy to prevent vomiting.

**Antigen**  Any substance not normally present in the body that stimulates the body to produce antibodies.

**Antihistamine**  A drug used to reduce effects associated with colds and allergies.

**Antineoplastics**  Drugs that prevent the growth and development of malignant cells.

**Antioxidant**  A substance that can protect another substance from oxidation; added to foods to keep oxygen from changing the food's color.

**Antispasmodic**  A drug used to relieve cramping and spasms of the stomach, intestines, and bladder.

**Antitoxin**  An antibody formed in response to—and capable of—neutralizing a poison of biologic origin.

**Aphrodisiac**  An agent that produces sexual desire.

**Apnea**  Temporary cessation of breathing, usually during sleep.

**Arthritis** Inflammation of joints.

**Assimilation** The process whereby nutrients are used by the body and changed into living tissue.

**Asthma** Condition of lungs characterized by a decrease in the diameter of some air passages; a spasm of the bronchial tubes or swelling of their mucous membranes.

**Ataxia** Loss of coordinated movement.

**Avidin** A protein in egg white capable of inactivating biotin.

**Bacteriophage** A virus that infects bacteria.

**Bariatrician** A weight-control doctor.

**BATF** Bureau of Alcohol, Tobacco, and Firearms.

**B-cells** White blood cells, made in the bone marrow, which produce antibodies on instructions from T-cells, white blood cells manufactured in the thymus.

**BHA** Butylated hydroxyanisole; a preservative and antioxidant used in many products; insoluble in water; can be toxic to the kidneys.

**BHT** Butylated hydroxytoluene; a solid, white crystalline antioxidant used to retard spoilage of many foods; can be more toxic to the kidneys than its nearly identical chemical cousin, BHA.

**Bioflavonoids** Citrus-flavored compounds necessary for healthy blood vessel walls; available in plants, citrus fruits, and rose hips; known as vitamin P-complex.

**BSE** Bovine spongiform encephalopathy; mad cow disease.

**Calciferol** A colorless, odorless crystalline material that is insoluble in water, soluble in fats; synthetic form of vitamin D.

**Calcium gluconate** An organic form of calcium.

**Carcinogen** A cancer-causing substance.

**Cardiac arrhythmia** Irregular heart action caused by disturbances in the discharge of cardiac impulses.

**Cardiovascular** Pertaining to heart and blood vessels.

**Carotene** An orange-yellow pigment in many plants that can be converted into vitamin A in the body.

**Casein** The protein in milk that has become the standard by which protein quality is measured.

**Catalyst** A substance that modifies (especially increases) the rate of chemical reaction without being consumed or changed in the process.

**Cataract** Clouding of the lens of the eye, which prevents clear vision.

**Cellulose** A fibrous, nondigestible carbohydrate; aids in intestinal elimination; provides no nutrient value.

**Chelation** A process by which mineral substances are changed into easily digestible form.

**Chronic** Of long duration; continuing; constant.

**Cirrhosis** A chronic liver disease characterized by dense or hardened connective tissue, degenerative changes, or alteration in structure.

**CJD** Creutzfeldt-Jakob disease; human variant of mad cow disease.

**CNS** Central nervous system.

**Coenzyme** The major portion, though nonprotein part, of an enzyme; usually a B vitamin.

**Colitis** Inflammation of the large intestine.

**Collagen** The primary organic constituent of bone, cartilage, and connective tissue.

**Congenital** Condition existing at birth; not hereditary.

**Corticosterone** An adrenal cortex hormone that influences the metabolism of carbohydrates, potassium, and sodium; essential for normal absorption of glucose.

**Cortisone** An adrenal gland hormone; also used as an anti-inflammatory agent.

**CPR** Cardiopulmonary resuscitation.

**Dehydration** A condition resulting from excessive loss of water from the body.

**Dermatitis** An inflammation of the skin; a rash.

**Desiccated** Dried; preserved by removing moisture.

**DHA** Docosahexaenoic acid; a member of the omega-3 family of essential fatty acids; made in the body from alpha-linolenic acid; found mainly in cold-water fish.

**Dicalcium phosphate** A filler used in pills that is derived from purified mineral rocks and is an excellent source of calcium and phosphorus.

**Diluents** Fillers; inert material added to tablets to increase their bulk in order to make them a practical size for compression.

**Diuretic** A substance that increases the output of urine from the body.

**DNA** Deoxyribonucleic acid; the nucleic acid in chromosomes that is part of the chemical basis for hereditary characteristics.

**DV** The percent Daily Value; used on food labels as recommendations for nutrients regardless of age or gender.

**Dyspepsia** Indigestion.

**EDB** Ethylene dibromide; a carcinogenic pesticide used to fumigate grain.

**Edema** Excessive accumulation of tissue fluid.

**Endogenous** Produced from within the body.

**EDTA** Ethylenediaminetetraacetic acid; a food additive that may have mutagenic or teratogenic properties.

**Enteritis** Inflammation of the intestines, particularly the small intestines.

**Enzyme** A protein substance found in living cells that brings about chemical changes; necessary for digestion of food.

**EPA** Environmental Protection Agency.

**Epidermis** The outer layer of skin.

**Epilepsy** Convulsive disorder.

**Estrogens** Female sex hormones.

**Excipient** Any inert substance used as a diluent or vehicle for a drug.

**Exogenous** Derived or developed from external causes.

**FBD** Fibrocystic breast disease, a common condition in which often painful, noncancerous cysts or lumps develop in the breast.

**FDA** Food and Drug Administration.

**Fibrin** An insoluble protein that forms the necessary fibrous network in the coagulation of blood.

**Free radicals** Uncontrolled oxidations that damage cells and weaken the immune system.

**Fructose** A natural sugar occurring in fruits and honey; often used as a preservative.

**Glucose** Blood sugar; a product of the body's assimilation of carbohydrates and a major source of energy.

**Glutamic acid** An amino acid present in all complete proteins; usually manufactured from vegetable protein; used as a salt substitute and a flavor-intensifying agent.

**Glutamine** An amino acid that constitutes, with glucose, the major nourishment used by the nervous system.

**Gluten** A mixture of two proteins—gliadin and glutenin—present in wheat, rye, oats, and barley.

**Glycogen** The body's chief storage carbohydrate, primarily stored in the liver.

**Gout** Upset in metabolism of uric acid, causing inflammation of joints, particularly in the knee or foot.

**GRAS** Generally Recognized As Safe.

**Half-life** The time it takes for half the amount of a drug to be metabolized or inactivated by the body (disappear from the bloodstream).

**HDL** High-density lipoprotein; carries fats and cholesterol through the bloodstream; considered the "good" cholesterol.

**Hepatitis** Inflammation of the liver.

**Hesperdin** Part of the C-complex.

**HFCS** High-fructose corn syrup.

**Holistic treatment** Treatment of the whole person.

**Homeostasis** The body's physiological equilibrium.

**Hormone** A substance formed in endocrine organs and transported by body fluids to activate other specifically receptive organs.

**HPP** Hydrolyzed plant protein; generally made from soybean or peanut meals. (See HVP.)

**Humectant** A substance that is used to preserve the moisture content of materials.

**HVP** Hydrolyzed vegetable protein; generally obtained from protein recovered from the wet milling of grains such as wheat and corn. Sometimes identified on labels as hydrolyzed cereal solids; components contain glutamic acid.

**Hydrochloric acid** A normally acidic part of the body's gastric juices.

**Hydrolyzed** Put into water-soluble form.

**Hydrolyzed protein chelate** Protein that is water soluble and chelated for easy assimilation.

**Hypertension** High blood pressure.

**Hypervitaminosis** A condition caused by an excessive ingestion of vitamins.

**Hypoglycemia** Low blood sugar.

**Hypotension** Low blood pressure.

**Hypovitaminosis** A deficiency disease resulting from an absence of vitamins in the diet.

**Idiopathic** A condition whose causes are not known.

**Immune** Protected against disease.

**Infectious** Likely to be transmitted by infection.

**Inflammation** Changes that occur in living tissues when invaded by germs; swelling, pain, and heat.

**Insulin** The hormone secreted by the pancreas that regulates the metabolism of sugar in the body.

**IU** International units.

**Jaundice** Increase in bile pigment in blood, causing a yellow tinge to skin, mucous membranes, and eyes; can be caused by disease of the liver, gallbladder, bile system, or blood.

**Lactating** Producing milk.

**Lactation** Secretion of milk by breasts.

**LAL** Lysinoalanine, a substance formed by the heating of casein, along with an alkali-treating process, that is suspected of causing kidney damage.

**Laxative** A substance that stimulates evacuation of the bowels.

**LDL** Low-density lipoprotein; the "bad" substance that deposits cholesterol along the artery walls when oxidized.

**Linoleic acid** One of the polyunsaturated fats, a constituent of lecithin; known as vitamin F; indispensable for life; must be obtained from foods.

**Lipfuscin** Age pigment in cells.

**Lipid** A fat or fatty substance.

**Lipotropic** Preventing abnormal or excessive accumulation of fat in the liver.

**Megavitamin therapy** Treatment of illness with massive amounts of vitamins.

**Menopause** Cessation of menstruation; usually between ages forty-five and fifty.

**Metabolize** To undergo change by physical and chemical processes.

**MUFA** Monounsaturated fatty acid.

**Narcotic** An addictive central nervous system depressant that blunts pain, distorts the senses, and induces sleep; may produce unconsciousness and death.

**Nausea** Stomach discomfort with the feeling of a need to vomit.

**Neuron** Nerve cell.

**Neurotransmitter** A chemical that transports messages between neurons in the brain.

**Nitrites** Substances used as fixatives in cured meats; can cause dangerous cancer-causing agents called nitrosamines.

**NLEA** Nutrition Labeling and Education Act of 1990.

**NSF** National Sanitation Foundation.

**Obesity** Excessive stoutness.

**Omega-3** A family of essential fatty acids generally supplied inadequately in the modern diet; the primary omega-3 is alpha-linolenic acid.

**Omega-6** A family of essential fatty acids abundant in the modern diet; the primary omega-6 is linolenic acid.

**Ophthalmic** Pertaining to eyes.

**Orthomolecular** The right molecule used for the right treatment; doctors who practice preventive medicine with vitamin therapies are called orthomolecular physicians.

**OSHA** Occupational Safety and Health Administration.

**Osteoporosis** A condition characterized by porous (softening or increasingly brittle) bones.

**Oxalates** Organic chemicals found in certain foods which can combine with calcium to form calcium oxalate, an insoluble chemical the body cannot use.

**PABA** Para-aminobenzoic acid; a component of the B-complex.

**Palmitate** Water-solubilized vitamin A.

**Parasite** Any animal or plant that lives inside or on the body of another animal or plant.

**PCBs** Polychlorinated biphenyls; toxic industrial-waste contaminants.

**PCRM** Physicians Committee for Responsible Medicine.

**Peptic** Pertaining to the digestive tract.

**pH** Degree of acidity or alkalinity of a substance.

**Photosensitivity** Sensitivity to light.

**PKU (phenylketonuria)** A hereditary disease caused by the lack of an enzyme needed to convert an essential amino acid (phenylalanine) into a form usable by the body; can cause mental retardation unless detected early in life.

**Polyunsaturated fats** Highly nonsaturated fats from vegetable sources; tend to lower blood cholesterol.

**PPM** Parts per million.

**Predigested protein** Protein that has been processed for fast assimilation to go directly into the bloodstream.

**Provitamin** A vitamin precursor; a chemical substance necessary to produce a vitamin.

**Psoriasis** A skin condition characterized by silver-scaled red patches.

**Psychosis** Type of insanity in which one almost completely loses touch with reality.

**PUFA** Polyunsaturated fatty acid.

**Radon** A naturally occurring form of radiation that seeps upward from the ground; carcinogenic.

**RDA** Recommended Dietary Allowances as established by the Food and Nutrition Board, National Academy of Sciences, and National Research Council.

**RDI** Reference Daily Intake; based on Recommended Dietary Allowances; used on labels as the percent Daily Value (DV).

**Rhinitis** Inflammation of the lining of the nose.

**RNA** Ribonucleic acid.

**Rose hips** A rich source of vitamin C; the nodule underneath the bud of a rose called a hip, in which the plant produces the vitamin C processors extract.

**Rutin** A substance extracted from buckwheat; part of the C-complex.

**Saturated fatty acids** Usually solid at room temperature; higher proportions found in foods from animal sources; tend to raise blood cholesterol levels.

**Sequestrant** A substance that absorbs ions and prevents changes that would affect the flavor, texture, and color of food; used for water softening.

**Soporific** Producing sleep.

**Steroid hormones** The sex hormones and hormones of the adrenal cortex.

**Steroids** A family of cortisone-like medications; prescribed when adrenal glands do not produce enough of the hormone cortisone; also used for treatment of swellings, allergic reactions, and other conditions.

**Sulfonamides** A group of sulfa drugs used to treat specific infections unresponsive to other antibacterials.

**Synergistic** The action of two or more substances to produce an effect that neither alone could accomplish.

**Synthetic** Produced artificially.

**Systemic** Pertaining to the whole body.

**T-cells** White blood cells, manufactured in the thymus, which protect the body from bacteria, viruses, and cancer-causing agents, while controlling the production of B-cells, which produce antibodies, and unwanted production of potentially harmful T-cells.

**Tachycardia** Rapid beating of the heart, coming on in sudden attacks.

**Teratogen** Anything that causes the development of abnormalities in an embryo.

**Tocopherols** The group of compounds (alpha, beta, delta, epsilon, eta, gamma, and zeta) that make vitamin E; obtained through the vacuum distillation of edible vegetable oils.

**Topical** Applied externally.

**Toxicity** The quality or condition of being poisonous, harmful, or destructive.

**Toxin** An organic poison produced in living or dead organisms.

**Trans-fatty acids** Artificial fatty acids produced by hydrogenation; although unsaturated, act like saturated fats and are unhealthy.

**Triglycerides** Fatty substances in the blood.

**Ulcer** Sore or lesion on skin surface or internal mucous membranes.

**Unsaturated fatty acids** Most often liquid at room temperature; primarily found in vegetable fats.

**USAN** United States Adopted Names Council; cosponsored by the American Pharmaceutical Association (APhA), American Medical Association (AMA), and United States Pharmacopia (USP) for the specific purpose of coining suitable, acceptable, nonproprietary names in the drug field.

**USRDA** United States Recommended Daily Allowances.

**Vasodilator** A drug that dilates (widens) blood vessels.

**Zein** Protein from corn.

**Zyme** A fermenting substance.

# Bibliography and Recommended Reading

TO THE NUTRITIONISTS, pharmacists, doctors, scientists, therapists, dieticians, researchers, government agencies, authors, and journalists whose works in the field of health and nutrition proved indispensable to the scope and completion of this book, I owe an enormous debt of gratitude.

The list that follows is provided to acknowledge my sincere and wholehearted appreciation to them, and to provide you with an opportunity for further reading in areas pertaining to your own particular interest of special medical and nutritional needs.

Acheson, Dr. David W. K., and Robin K. Levinson. *Safe Eating*. New York: Dell Publishing, 1998.

Barnes, Julian E., and Greg Winter. "Stressed Out? Bad Knee? Relief Promised in a Juice." *New York Times* (May 27, 2001).

Bricklin, Mark. *Prevention Magazine's Nutrition Advisor*. Emmaus, PA: Rodale Press, 1993.

Brody, Jane E. "Clean Cutting Boards Are Not Enough: New Lessons in Food Safety." *New York Times* (January 30, 2001).

———. "The Culprits, When Good Food Goes Bad." *New York Times* (February 6, 2001).

Brown, Kathryn. "Seeds of Concern." *Scientific American* (April 2001).

Center for Science in the Public Interest. *Nutrition Action Health Letter* (March 1999).

Cody, Dr. Mildred M. *Safe Food for You and Your Family.* New York: John Wiley & Sons, 1996.

*Consumer Reports.* "It's Only Water, Right?" (August 2000).

Cook, Kenneth A. "How to Protect Yourself from Pesticides in Your Food." *Bottom Line* (April 15, 1999).

Cowley, Geoffrey. "Cannibals to Cows: The Path of a Deadly Disease." *Newsweek* (March 12, 2001).

Dewall, Caroline Smith, Lucy Alderton, and Bonnie Liebman. "Food Safety Guide." *Nutrition Action Health Letter* 26, no. 8 (October 1999).

Dominus, Susan. "The Allergy Prison." *New York Times Magazine* (June 10, 2001).

Duffy, William. *Sugar Blues.* New York: Warner Books, 1993.

Fox, Nicols. *It Was Probably Something You Ate: A Practical Guide to Avoiding and Surviving Foodborne Illness.* New York: Penguin, 1999.

Gittleman, Ann Louise. *Get the Sugar Out: 501 Simple Ways to Cut the Sugar in Any Diet.* New York: Crown Publishing, 1996.

Glausiusz, Josin. "Can You Stomach It?" *Discover Magazine* (March 2001).

Hale, Ellen. "Britain Takes Lead in Fighting Mad Cow Disease." *USA Today* (December 6, 2000).

Jacobson, Dr. Michael F., Lisa Y. Lefferts, and Anne Witte Garland. *Safe Food.* Los Angeles: Living Planet Press, 1991.

Johnson, Sharlene K. "Pesticides: What You Don't Know Can Hurt You." *Ladies Home Journal* (June 1997).

Knight, Jan. "Good from the Ground Up?" *Herbs for Health* (March/April 2000).

———. "Soy Meets World." *Herbs for Health* (November/December 2000).

Kolata, Gina. "Putting a Price Tag on the Priceless." *New York Times* (April 8, 2001).

Kulman, Linda. "Pregnant Women Get No Bologna—or Shark or Brie." *U.S. News & World Report* (January 29, 2001).

———. "Steakhouse Craze Defies Healthful Eating Edict." *U.S. News & World Report* (March 12, 2001).

Kunzig, Robert. "Chemistry of Plastics." *Discover Magazine* (December 2000).

Lapchick, Michael J., et al. *The Label Reader's Pocket Dictionary of Food Additives: A Comprehensive Quick Reference Guide to More Than 250 of Today's Common Food Additives.* New York: John Wiley & Sons, 1993.

Liebman, Bonnie. "Dioxin for Dinner?" *Nutrition Action Newsletter* (October 2000).

Loken, Joan K. *The HACCP Food Safety Manual.* New York: John Wiley & Sons, 1995.

Lowe, Cari. "The Joys of Soy: Nature's Little Cancer Fighter." *Health Products Business* (February 2001).

Mandile, Maria Noel. "Warning for Tea and Coffee Drinkers." *Natural Health Magazine* (April 2001).

Miller, Sue. "A Natural Mood Booster." *Newsweek* (May 5, 1997).

Mindell, Earl. *Earl Mindell's Anti-Aging Bible.* New York: Fireside, 1996.

———. *Earl Mindell's Herb Bible.* New York: Fireside, 1992.

———. *Earl Mindell's Soy Miracle.* New York: Fireside, 1995.

———. *Earl Mindell's Vitamin Bible for the 21st Century.* New York: Warner Books, 1999.

Osborne, Sally Eauclaire. "Does Soy Have a Dark Side?" *Natural Health* (March 1999).

Pennington, Jean A.T., Ph.D., et al. *Bowed and Church's Food Values of Portions Commonly Used.* 17th ed. New York: Lippincott, 1997.

Pollack, Andrew. "The Green Revolution Yields to the Bottom Line." *New York Times* (May 15, 2001).

Pollan, Michael. "Naturally." *New York Times Magazine* (May 13, 2001).

Rebhahn, Peter. "Dangerous Diet Drinks." *Psychology Today* (March/April 2001).

Robertson, Joel C., and Tom Monte (contrib.). *Natural Prozac: Learning to Release Your Body's Own Anti-Depressants.* New York: HarperCollins, 1998.

Rudin, Donald O., and Clara Felix. *Omega-3 Oils: To Improve Mental Health, Fight Degenerative Diseases, and Extend Your Life.* New York: Avery Penguin Putnam, 1996.

Rue, Nancy, Richard Linton, and David Zachery McSwane. *Essentials of Food Safety.* New York: Prentice Hall, 2000.

Schardt, David. "Food Allergies." *Nutrition Action Healthletter* (April 2001).

Schlosser, Eric. *Fast Food Nation.* Boston: Houghton Mifflin Co., 2001.

Schnoor, Jerald L. *Environmental Modeling: Fate and Transport of Pollutants in Water, Air, and Soil.* New York: John Wiley & Sons, 1996.

Scott, Elizabeth, and Paul Sockett. *How to Prevent Food Poisoning.* New York: John Wiley & Sons, 1998.

Sinopoulus, Artemis P., M.D., and Jo Robinson. *The Omega Plan*. New York: HarperCollins, 1998.

Steinman, David. *Diet for a Poisoned Planet*. New York: Harmony Books, 1990.

Steward, Leighton H., et al. *Sugar Busters! Cut Sugar to Trim Fat*. New York: Ballantine Books, 1998.

Ticciati, Laura, and Robin Ticciati. *Genetically Engineered Foods: Are They Safe? You Decide*. New York: McGraw-Hill, 1998.

Tyler, Varro E., Ph.D. "The Truth About FDA Approval." *Prevention* (June 2001).

Uehling, Mark D. "Farms or Pharmacies?" *Popular Science* (August 1999).

Wheelwright, Jeff. "Who's Minding the Store." *Discover Magazine* (March 2001).

Wichman, Larry. "Foods That Kill." *Men's Fitness* (October 1999).

Williams, Rose Marie, M.A. "Plastics: The Sixth Basic Food Group—Part 2." *Townsend Letter for Doctors & Patients* (February/March 2001).

Winter, Greg. "Contaminated Food Sickens Millions Despite Advances." *New York Times* (March 3, 2001).

Winter, Ruth. *A Consumer's Dictionary of Food Additives*. 5th ed. New York: Three Rivers Press, 1999.

———. *Poisons in Your Food: The Dangers You Face and What You Can Do About Them*. New York: Crown Publishing, 1991.

Wood, Rebecca. *The New Whole Foods Encyclopedia: A Comprehensive Resource for Healthy Eating*. New York: Penguin, 1999.

Wotecki, Catherine E., and Paul R. Thomas (eds.). *Eat for Life: The Food and Nutrition Board's Guide to Reducing Your Risk of Chronic Disease*. Washington, DC: National Academy Press, 1992.

Zitner, Aaron. "Gene-Altered Catfish Raise Environmental, Legal Issues." *Los Angeles Times* (January 2, 2001).

# Index